# Financing and Payment Strategies to Support High-Quality Care for People with Serious Illness

## PROCEEDINGS OF A WORKSHOP

Laurene Graig, Elaine Soohoo, and Joe Alper, *Rapporteurs*

Roundtable on Quality Care for People with Serious Illness

Board on Health Care Services

Board on Health Sciences Policy

Health and Medicine Division

*The National Academies of*
SCIENCES · ENGINEERING · MEDICINE

THE NATIONAL ACADEMIES PRESS
*Washington, DC*
**www.nap.edu**

THE NATIONAL ACADEMIES PRESS  500 Fifth Street, NW  Washington, DC 20001

This activity was supported by contract No. HHSN263201200074I (Task Order No. HHSN26300096) with the National Institute of Nursing Research/National Institutes of Health and by Aetna Inc., Altarum Institute, American Academy of Hospice and Palliative Medicine, American Cancer Society, American Geriatrics Society, Anthem, Inc., Ascension Health, Association of Professional Chaplains, Association of Rehabilitation Nurses, Blue Cross Blue Shield Association, Blue Cross Blue Shield of Massachusetts, California State University Institute for Palliative Care, Cambia Health Solutions, Cedars-Sinai Health System, Center to Advance Palliative Care, Centers for Medicare & Medicaid Services, Coalition to Transform Advanced Care, Common Practice, Excellus BlueCross BlueShield, Federation of American Hospitals, The Greenwall Foundation, Hospice and Palliative Nurses Association, The John A. Hartford Foundation, Kaiser Permanente, Gordon and Betty Moore Foundation, National Coalition for Hospice and Palliative Care, National Hospice and Palliative Care Organization, National Palliative Care Research Center, National Patient Advocate Foundation, National Quality Forum, Oncology Nursing Society, Patient-Centered Outcomes Research Institute, Sentara Healthcare, Social Work Hospice and Palliative Care Network, Supportive Care Coalition, Susan G. Komen, UnitedHealth Group, and the National Academy of Medicine. Any opinions, findings, conclusions, or recommendations expressed in this publication do not necessarily reflect the views of any organization or agency that provided support for the project.

International Standard Book Number-13:  978-0-309-47444-3
International Standard Book Number-10:  0-309-47444-2
Digital Object Identifier:  https://doi.org/10.17226/25071

Additional copies of this publication are available for sale from the National Academies Press, 500 Fifth Street, NW, Keck 360, Washington, DC 20001; (800) 624-6242 or (202) 334-3313; http://www.nap.edu.

Copyright 2018 by the National Academy of Sciences. All rights reserved.

Printed in the United States of America

Suggested citation: National Academies of Sciences, Engineering, and Medicine. 2018. *Financing and payment strategies to support high-quality care for people with serious illness: Proceedings of a workshop.* Washington, DC: The National Academies Press. doi: https://doi.org/10.17226/25071.

# The National Academies of
## SCIENCES · ENGINEERING · MEDICINE

The **National Academy of Sciences** was established in 1863 by an Act of Congress, signed by President Lincoln, as a private, nongovernmental institution to advise the nation on issues related to science and technology. Members are elected by their peers for outstanding contributions to research. Dr. Marcia McNutt is president.

The **National Academy of Engineering** was established in 1964 under the charter of the National Academy of Sciences to bring the practices of engineering to advising the nation. Members are elected by their peers for extraordinary contributions to engineering. Dr. C. D. Mote, Jr., is president.

The **National Academy of Medicine** (formerly the Institute of Medicine) was established in 1970 under the charter of the National Academy of Sciences to advise the nation on medical and health issues. Members are elected by their peers for distinguished contributions to medicine and health. Dr. Victor J. Dzau is president.

The three Academies work together as the **National Academies of Sciences, Engineering, and Medicine** to provide independent, objective analysis and advice to the nation and conduct other activities to solve complex problems and inform public policy decisions. The National Academies also encourage education and research, recognize outstanding contributions to knowledge, and increase public understanding in matters of science, engineering, and medicine.

Learn more about the National Academies of Sciences, Engineering, and Medicine at **www.nationalacademies.org**.

*The National Academies of*
SCIENCES • ENGINEERING • MEDICINE

**Consensus Study Reports** published by the National Academies of Sciences, Engineering, and Medicine document the evidence-based consensus on the study's statement of task by an authoring committee of experts. Reports typically include findings, conclusions, and recommendations based on information gathered by the committee and the committee's deliberations. Each report has been subjected to a rigorous and independent peer-review process and it represents the position of the National Academies on the statement of task.

**Proceedings** published by the National Academies of Sciences, Engineering, and Medicine chronicle the presentations and discussions at a workshop, symposium, or other event convened by the National Academies. The statements and opinions contained in proceedings are those of the participants and are not endorsed by other participants, the planning committee, or the National Academies.

For information about other products and activities of the National Academies, please visit www.nationalacademies.org/about/whatwedo.

## PLANNING COMMITTEE FOR A WORKSHOP ON FINANCING AND PAYMENT STRATEGIES TO SUPPORT HIGH-QUALITY CARE FOR PEOPLE WITH SERIOUS ILLNESS[1]

**MARK B. GANZ** (*Co-Chair*), President and Chief Executive Officer, Cambia Health Solutions
**HAIDEN HUSKAMP** (*Co-Chair*), 30th Anniversary Professor of Health Care Policy, Harvard Medical School
**ROBERT A. BERGAMINI,** Medical Director, Palliative Care Services, Mercy Clinic Children's Cancer and Hematology, representing the Supportive Care Coalition
**PATRICIA A. BOMBA,** Vice President and Medical Director, Geriatrics, Excellus BlueCross BlueShield
**STEPHEN FRIEDHOFF,** Senior Vice President, Clinical Strategy and Programs, Anthem, Inc.
**LEE GOLDBERG,** Director, Improving End-of-Life Care Project, The Pew Charitable Trusts
**ANNA GOSLINE,** Senior Director of Health Policy and Strategic Initiatives, Blue Cross Blue Shield of Massachusetts
**ZIAD HAYDAR,** Senior Vice President and Chief Clinical Officer, Ascension Health
**JOANNE LYNN,** Director, Center for Elder Care and Advanced Illness, Altarum Institute
**JAMES MITTELBERGER,** Director and Chief Medical Officer, Optum Center for Palliative and Supportive Care, UnitedHealth Group (*through July 2017*)
**SHARON SCRIBNER PEARCE,** Vice President, Policy, National Hospice and Palliative Care Organization
**LEONARD D. SCHAEFFER,** Judge Robert Maclay Widney Chair and Professor, University of Southern California
**ALLISON SILVERS,** Vice President for Payment and Policy, Center to Advance Palliative Care

---

[1] The National Academies of Sciences, Engineering, and Medicine's planning committees are solely responsible for organizing the workshop, identifying topics, and choosing speakers. The responsibility for the published Proceedings of a Workshop rests with the workshop rapporteurs and the institution.

*Project Staff*

**LAURENE GRAIG,** Director, Roundtable on Quality Care for People with Serious Illness
**SYLARA MARIE CRUZ,** Research Assistant
**SHARYL NASS,** Director, Board on Health Care Services, and Director, National Cancer Policy Forum
**ANDREW M. POPE,** Director, Board on Health Sciences Policy

*Consultant*

**JOE ALPER,** Consulting Writer

# ROUNDTABLE ON QUALITY CARE FOR PEOPLE WITH SERIOUS ILLNESS[1]

**LEONARD D. SCHAEFFER** (*Chair*), Judge Robert Maclay Widney Chair and Professor, University of Southern California

**JAMES A. TULSKY** (*Vice Chair*), Chair, Department of Psychosocial Oncology and Palliative Care, Dana-Farber Cancer Institute; Chief, Division of Palliative Medicine, Brigham and Women's Hospital; Professor of Medicine and Co-Director, Center for Palliative Care, Harvard Medical School

**JENNIFER BALLENTINE,** Executive Director, California State University Institute for Palliative Care

**ROBERT A. BERGAMINI,** Medical Director, Palliative Care Services, Mercy Clinic Children's Cancer and Hematology, representing the Supportive Care Coalition

**AMY J. BERMAN,** Senior Program Officer, The John A. Hartford Foundation

**PATRICIA A. BOMBA,** Vice President and Medical Director, Geriatrics, Excellus BlueCross BlueShield

**GRACE B. CAMPBELL,** Assistant Professor, Department of Acute and Tertiary Care, University of Pittsburgh School of Nursing, representing the Association of Rehabilitation Nurses

**STEVE CLAUSER,** Program Director, Improving Healthcare Systems, Patient-Centered Outcomes Research Institute

**JEFF COHN,** Medical Director, Common Practice

**JANET CORRIGAN,** Chief Program Officer, Patient Care Program, Gordon and Betty Moore Foundation

**ANDREW DREYFUS,** President and Chief Executive Officer, Blue Cross Blue Shield of Massachusetts

**CAROLE REDDING FLAMM,** Executive Medical Director, Blue Cross Blue Shield Association

**STEPHEN FRIEDHOFF,** Senior Vice President, Clinical Strategy and Programs, Anthem, Inc.

**MARK B. GANZ,** President and Chief Executive Officer, Cambia Health Solutions

---

[1] The National Academies of Sciences, Engineering, and Medicine's forums and roundtables do not issue, review, or approve individual documents. The responsibility for the published Proceedings of a Workshop rests with the workshop rapporteurs and the institution.

**ZIAD HAYDAR,** Senior Vice President and Chief Clinical Officer, Ascension Health

**PAMELA S. HINDS,** Director of Nursing Research and Quality Outcomes, Children's National Health System

**HAIDEN HUSKAMP,** 30th Anniversary Professor of Health Care Policy, Harvard Medical School

**KIMBERLY JOHNSON,** Associate Professor of Medicine, Senior Fellow in the Center for the Study of Aging and Human Development, Duke University School of Medicine

**CHARLES N. KAHN III,** President and Chief Executive Officer, Federation of American Hospitals

**REBECCA A. KIRCH,** Executive Vice President of Healthcare Quality and Value, National Patient Advocate Foundation

**TOM KOUTSOUMPAS,** Co-Founder, Coalition to Transform Advanced Care

**SHARI M. LING,** Deputy Chief Medical Officer, Centers for Medicare & Medicaid Services

**BERNARD LO,** President and Chief Executive Officer, The Greenwall Foundation

**JOANNE LYNN,** Director, Center for Elder Care and Advanced Illness, Altarum Institute

**DIANE E. MEIER,** Director, Center to Advance Palliative Care

**AMY MELNICK,** Executive Director, National Coalition for Hospice and Palliative Care

**JERI L. MILLER,** Chief, Office of End-of-Life and Palliative Care Research, National Institute of Nursing Research, National Institutes of Health

**R. SEAN MORRISON,** Director, National Palliative Care Research Center

**MURALI NAIDU,** Vice President, Chief Clinical Officer, Sentara Healthcare

**BRENDA NEVIDJON,** Chief Executive Officer, Oncology Nursing Society

**HAROLD L. PAZ,** Executive Vice President and Chief Medical Officer, Aetna Inc.

**SHARON SCRIBNER PEARCE,** Vice President, Policy, National Hospice and Palliative Care Organization

**JUDITH R. PERES,** Long-Term and Palliative Care Consultant, Clinical Social Worker, and Board Member, Social Work Hospice and Palliative Care Network

**PHILLIP A. PIZZO,** Founding Director, Stanford Distinguished Careers Institute; former Dean, Stanford School of Medicine and David and Susan Heckerman Professor of Pediatrics and of Microbiology and Immunology

**WENDY PRINS,** Senior Advisor, Quality Innovation, National Quality Forum

**THOMAS M. PRISELAC,** President and Chief Executive Officer, Cedars-Sinai Health System

**JOANNE REIFSNYDER,** Executive Vice President, Clinical Operations and Chief Nursing Officer, Genesis Healthcare, representing the Hospice and Palliative Nurses Association

**JUDITH A. SALERNO,** President, The New York Academy of Medicine

**KATRINA M. SCOTT,** Oncology Chaplain, Massachusetts General Hospital, representing the Association of Professional Chaplains

**KATHERINE SHARPE,** Senior Vice President, Patient and Caregiver Support, American Cancer Society

**JOSEPH W. SHEGA,** Regional Medical Director, VITAS Hospice Care, representing the American Geriatrics Society

**CHRISTIAN SINCLAIR,** Outpatient Palliative Oncology Lead, Division of Palliative Medicine, University of Kansas Health System, representing the American Academy of Hospice and Palliative Medicine

**TANYA STEWART,** Senior Medical Director, UnitedHealthcare Retiree Solutions

**SUSAN ELIZABETH WANG,** Regional Lead for Shared Decision-Making and Advance Care Planning, Southern California Permanente Medical Group, Kaiser Permanente

*Roundtable on Quality Care for People with Serious Illness Staff*

**LAURENE GRAIG,** Director, Roundtable on Quality Care for People with Serious Illness
**SYLARA MARIE CRUZ,** Research Assistant
**PATRICK BURKE,** Financial Associate

**ELAINE SOOHOO,** Christine Mirzayan Science & Technology Policy Graduate Fellow (*January–April 2018*)
**SHARYL NASS,** Director, Board on Health Care Services, and Director, National Cancer Policy Forum
**ANDREW M. POPE,** Director, Board on Health Sciences Policy

# Reviewers

This Proceedings of a Workshop was reviewed in draft form by individuals chosen for their diverse perspectives and technical expertise. The purpose of this independent review is to provide candid and critical comments that will assist the National Academies of Sciences, Engineering, and Medicine in making each published proceedings as sound as possible and to ensure that it meets the institutional standards for quality, objectivity, evidence, and responsiveness to the charge. The review comments and draft manuscript remain confidential to protect the integrity of the process.

We thank the following individuals for their review of this proceedings:

**EMILY CHAI,** Mount Sinai School of Medicine
**JEANNE CHIRICO,** Hospice & Palliative Care Association of New York State
**TORRIE FIELDS,** Blue Shield of California
**ROBERT FINE,** Baylor Scott and White Health
**VICKI JACKSON,** Harvard Medical School

Although the reviewers listed above provided many constructive comments and suggestions, they were not asked to endorse the content of the proceedings nor did they see the final draft before its release. The review of this proceedings was overseen by **BETTY FERRELL,** City of Hope National Medical Center. She was responsible for making certain that an independent examination of this proceedings was carried out in accordance with standards of the National Academies and that all review comments were carefully considered. Responsibility for the final content rests entirely with the rapporteurs and the National Academies.

# Acknowledgments

The National Academies of Sciences, Engineering, and Medicine's Roundtable on Quality Care for People with Serious Illness wishes to express its sincere gratitude to the Planning Committee Co-Chairs Mark Ganz and Haiden Huskamp for their valuable contributions to the development of this workshop. We also wish to thank all the members of the planning committee, who collaborated to ensure a workshop complete with informative presentations and rich discussions. We are extremely grateful to the speakers and moderators, who generously shared their expertise and their time with workshop participants.

Support from the many annual sponsors of the Roundtable on Quality Care for People with Serious Illness is critical to the roundtable's work. The sponsors include Aetna Inc., Altarum Institute, American Academy of Hospice and Palliative Medicine, American Cancer Society, American Geriatrics Society, Anthem, Inc., Ascension Health, Association of Professional Chaplains, Association of Rehabilitation Nurses, Blue Cross Blue Shield Association, Blue Cross Blue Shield of Massachusetts, California State University Institute for Palliative Care, Cambia Health Solutions, Cedars-Sinai Health System, Center to Advance Palliative Care, Centers for Medicare & Medicaid Services, Coalition to Transform Advanced Care, Common Practice, Excellus BlueCross BlueShield, Federation of American Hospitals, The Greenwall Foundation, Hospice and Palliative Nurses Association, The John A. Hartford Foundation, Kaiser Permanente,

Gordon and Betty Moore Foundation, National Coalition for Hospice and Palliative Care, National Hospice and Palliative Care Organization, National Institute of Nursing Research, National Palliative Care Research Center, National Patient Advocate Foundation, National Quality Forum, Oncology Nursing Society, Patient-Centered Outcomes Research Institute, Sentara Healthcare, Social Work Hospice and Palliative Care Network, Supportive Care Coalition, Susan G. Komen, UnitedHealth Group, and the National Academy of Medicine.

# Contents

ACRONYMS AND ABBREVIATIONS     xix

INTRODUCTION     1
PATIENT–CAREGIVER–CLINICIAN PERSPECTIVE ON
MANAGING AND PAYING FOR SERIOUS ILLNESS CARE     8
FRAMING THE CHALLENGES AND OPPORTUNITES FOR
FINANCING AND PAYMENT INNOVATION     12
    Taking Care of a Seriously Ill Patient in the Context of the
       Current Health Care Financing System, 18
    Discussion, 20
EXPLORING FINANCING AND PAYMENT INNOVATIONS:
CHALLENGES, IMPACTS, AND LESSONS FROM FEE-FOR-
SERVICE AND VALUE-BASED PAYMENT ARRANGEMENTS     23
    Financing Serious Illness Care at Cambia Health Solutions, 24
    CompassionNet: Community-Based Pediatric Palliative Care, 26
    Anthem's Enhanced Personal Health Care, 28
    Lessons from CMS Demonstration Projects, 31
    BSWH's Journey Toward Value in Serious Illness Care, 34
    Discussion, 36
VIEW FROM CONGRESS     38

EXPLORING FINANCING AND PAYMENT INNOVATIONS:
CHALLENGES, IMPACTS, AND LESSONS FROM GLOBAL
BUDGETING ARRANGEMENTS 40
    Financing Quality Care for Serious Illness at Kaiser Permanente, 40
    Global Payment Arrangements for Serious Illness Care in
        Massachusetts, 43
    Complex Care Management at OptumHealth, 47
    Discussion, 50
EXPLORING POTENTIAL REGULATORY AND POLICY
CHANGES TO ENSURE HIGH-QUALITY CARE FOR
PEOPLE OF ALL AGES WITH SERIOUS ILLNESS 52
    Policy Opportunities, 54
    Panel Discussion, 58
    Closing Thoughts, 62
REFERENCES 63

APPENDIX A: STATEMENT OF TASK 67
APPENDIX B: WORKSHOP AGENDA 69

# Box, Figures, and Table

**BOX**

1   Suggestions Made by Individual Workshop Participants Related to Finance and Payment Strategies for High-Quality Care for People with Serious Illness, 4

**FIGURES**

1   Distribution of out-of-pocket spending in the last 5 years of life, 14
2   Deaths at home by age, 27
3   Share of regional Medicare beneficiaries cared for under the Medicare Share Savings ACO program, 44
4   Share of members whose care was paid for under a global payment arrangement, 44

**TABLE**

1   Cost and Location of Death at Five Moments in the Last Year of Life, 29

# Acronyms and Abbreviations

| | |
|---|---|
| ACA | Patient Protection and Affordable Care Act of 2010 |
| ACO | accountable care organization |
| AQC | Alternative Quality Contract |
| | |
| BCBSMA | Blue Cross Blue Shield of Massachusetts |
| BCBSNC | Blue Cross Blue Shield of North Carolina |
| BPCI | Bundled Payments for Care Improvement |
| BSWH | Baylor Scott & White Health |
| | |
| CHIP | Children's Health Insurance Program |
| CHRONIC | Creating High-Quality Results and Outcomes Necessary to Improve Chronic Care Act |
| CMMI | Center for Medicare & Medicaid Innovation |
| CMS | Centers for Medicare & Medicaid Services |
| COBRA | Consolidated Omnibus Budget Reconciliation Act |
| COPD | chronic obstructive pulmonary disease |
| CPC Plus | Comprehensive Primary Care Plus |
| | |
| EHR | electronic health record |
| | |
| HEDIS | Healthcare Effectiveness Data and Information Set |

| | |
|---|---|
| I-SNP | Institutional Special Needs Plan |
| IMPACT | Improving Medicare Post-Acute Care Transformation Act of 2014 |
| MACRA | Medicare Access and Children's Health Insurance Program Reauthorization Act of 2015 |
| NCQA | National Committee for Quality Assurance |
| OECD | Organisation for Economic Co-operation and Development |
| PACE | Programs of All-Inclusive Care for the Elderly |
| PPO | preferred provider organization |
| SNF | skilled nursing facility |
| SNP | special needs plan |

# Proceedings of a Workshop

## INTRODUCTION[1]

Millions of people in the United States live with serious illnesses such as cancer, heart disease, chronic obstructive pulmonary disease (COPD), amyotrophic lateral sclerosis, Parkinson's disease, and dementia—often for many years. Those facing serious illness have a range of interconnected medical and non-medical needs, and the way their care is financed has a large impact on the care they receive. Medicare is the predominant payer, but both Medicaid and private payers also play significant roles in financing care for serious illness. In an effort to address the complex needs of people with serious illness, public and private health care payers are testing innovative financing strategies and alternative payment models. These innovative approaches signal a gradual transition from the traditional fee-for-service system that pays providers based on the quantity of services to a system based on the value of care provided and a heightened focus on improved quality of care at lower cost.

---

[1] The planning committee's role was limited to planning the workshop, and the Proceedings of a Workshop was prepared by the workshop rapporteurs as a factual summary of what occurred at the workshop. Statements, recommendations, and opinions expressed are those of individual presenters and participants, and are not necessarily endorsed or verified by the National Academies of Sciences, Engineering, and Medicine, and they should not be construed as reflecting any group consensus.

To explore this evolving financing and payment landscape for serious illness care within public- and private-sector programs, the Roundtable on Quality Care for People with Serious Illness developed a workshop, Financing and Payment Strategies to Support High-Quality Care for People with Serious Illness. The workshop was held on November 29, 2017, at the National Academies of Sciences, Engineering, and Medicine's Keck Center in Washington, DC. The workshop convened clinicians, researchers, policy analysts, and patient advocates, as well as representatives from academia, government and private health care plans, and insurers to discuss challenges and opportunities in financing high-quality care for people with serious illness.

As was discussed in a previous roundtable-sponsored workshop, there are proven models of caring for individuals living with serious illness that allow patients to be cared for at home, thus avoiding costly hospitalizations (NASEM, 2017b).[2] A key challenge, however, is developing financing and payment strategies to support those models nationwide. Compounding that challenge is the fact that many comprehensive approaches to serious illness care include services that often fall outside of those reimbursed by public and private plans, such as supportive services in the home or the community.

The Roundtable on Quality Care for People with Serious Illness serves to convene stakeholders from government, academia, industry, professional associations, nonprofit advocacy groups, and philanthropies. Inspired by and expanding on the work of the 2014 Institute of Medicine (IOM) consensus report *Dying in America: Improving Quality and Honoring Individual Preferences Near the End of Life* (IOM, 2015),[3] the roundtable aims to foster ongoing dialogue about crucial policy and research issues to accelerate and sustain progress in care for people of all ages experiencing serious illness.

In his introductory remarks to the workshop, Mark Ganz, president and chief executive officer of Cambia Health Solutions, noted that this was the third in a series of workshops focusing on the topic of how the nation can better care for those with serious illness. The first workshop introduced

---

[2] While opinion polls indicate a majority of patients prefer to be cared for at home, it is important to recognize that this is not always feasible, particularly for patients with dementia and acute care needs.

[3] As of March 2016, the Health and Medicine Division of the National Academies of Sciences, Engineering, and Medicine continues the consensus studies and convening activities previously carried out by the Institute of Medicine. The IOM name is used to refer to publications issued prior to July 2015.

the patient and caregiver voices (NASEM, 2017a), and Ganz reminded the workshop attendees that this is the place where this work must start, given that the goal is to make the journey "through health and sickness as straight and smooth and seamless" as possible for individuals and families dealing with serious illness. The second workshop focused on integrating principles of palliative care into care delivery models based on a deep understanding of what patients, their families, and their caregivers need and want (NASEM, 2017b). Ganz added that it was a natural progression for this workshop to discuss finance and payment strategies to support high-quality care for people with serious illness.

The workshop format began with an interview of a patient-caregiver and clinician, followed by moderated panel presentations, keynote addresses from members of Congress, and interactive audience discussion exploring a range of issues, including

- Gaps, challenges, and opportunities for innovative payment approaches to support high-quality care for people with serious illness;
- Approaches for innovation in fee-for-service and value-based payment and global-budgeting arrangements across a range of settings and populations;
- Lessons learned and key barriers identified from efforts to implement innovative financing and payment arrangements;
- Legislative environment regarding care for people with serious illness; and
- Insights on policy changes necessary at the federal and state levels to address barriers to financing and payment innovation to support high-quality care for people with serious illness.

Ganz pointed out that financing and payment are only part of the equation of high-quality care. "One thing to keep in mind as we go through the day is that sometimes we make a mistake in health care policy where we say that the way to solve a problem is to just figure out some way to pay for it," and that approach "can often lead to paying for things that actually are not improving the lives of individuals and their families," Ganz cautioned.

The workshop's first session featured the perspectives of a patient, who also became a caregiver to his seriously ill wife, and their clinician. This narrative served as a powerful illustration of the financial impact of serious illness on individuals and their families. The second half of the first session framed the challenges and opportunities for financing and payment innovation. The second session explored the lessons learned from examples of innovation in financing and payment in both fee-for-service and value-based payment frameworks. The workshop's luncheon session featured remarks by two members of Congress, who provided their perspectives on the legislative and policy environment as it relates to paying for high-quality serious illness care.

The afternoon sessions began with a panel that explored the challenges and opportunities for innovation in global budgeting arrangements and the barriers to innovation. The final session provided further insights and perspectives on policy and regulatory changes to ensure high-quality care for people with serious illness, followed by a discussion of the policy changes necessary at federal and state levels to address barriers to innovation in payment and financing that would better support individuals with serious illness.

This Proceedings of a Workshop summarizes the presentations and discussions. The speakers, panelists, and workshop participants presented a broad range of views and ideas. Box 1 provides a summary of suggestions

---

**BOX 1**
**Suggestions Made by Individual Workshop Participants Related to Finance and Payment Strategies for High-Quality Care for People with Serious Illness**

**Developing Innovative Financing and Policy Approaches to Support Comprehensive and Integrated Serious Illness Care**

- Consider financing plans that incorporate more social services and allow for a more integrated approach that encompasses a patient's physical, psychological, supportive, and spiritual needs. (Arakelian, Harris, Peres, Stevenson, Wang)
- Consider ways to change Medicare's financing system to a more integrated system, one that matches interconnected needs and considers the total cost of care, rather than a piecemeal approach that does not incentivize coordination of care. (Banach, Berman, Stevenson)

**BOX 1 Continued**

- Develop a network of community-based organizations that directly receive funds to provide needed services instead of having them trickle down from the acute care system. (Chirico)
- Include a hospice and palliative care benefit in integrated financing and delivery demonstrations. (Stevenson)
- Encourage state and local entities and health care systems to take the lead in developing innovative programs that improve quality, accessibility, and affordability and go beyond what the Centers for Medicare & Medicaid Services (CMS) would normally pay for, which are individual fee-for-service encounters for individual conditions. (Conway, Fine, Ling)
- Examine the structural relationship between Medicare and Medicaid to reduce or eliminate the inefficiencies resulting from a failure to coordinate available benefits more effectively under these two programs. (Banach)
- Recognize that the broader set of social services, long-term services, and supports wrapped around patients or members with complex conditions are often disconnected. Create a system that will more effectively connect those services. (Fine, Harris)
- Develop policy to create a bundle of supports and services that would help prevent decline in Medicare beneficiaries rather than having to wait for them to decline before providing care. (Banach)
- Build an evidence base that provides specific non-medical benefits to specific groups of beneficiaries; this will have a measurable effect on health outcomes and on the total cost of care. (Harris)
- Coordinate patient-centered care to produce the best outcomes for these individuals, as individuals with serious illness are more likely to experience transitions in care. (James, Wang)
- Develop specific payment models focused on serious illness care. (Conway)
- Develop policy to enable venture-backed companies that are trying to disrupt the Medicare fee-for-service space to have their models brought to scale if they prove to be effective. (Harris)

*continued*

**BOX 1 Continued**

- Build momentum that will last from one administration to the next by establishing state-based innovation across Medicare and Medicaid that can flow seamlessly across state lines. (Conway)

**Improving Quality by Focusing on What Is Being Measured and How Measures Are Used**

- Measure the impact of value-based care for serious illness on patient and family finances, in addition to direct health care costs, to see if such models shift more of the cost of care to patients and their families. (Morrison)
- Align financial incentives with accountability to ensure that value-based approaches do not result in diminished quality of care. (Stevenson)
- Use combined beneficiary and caregiver costs as the unit for cost analysis related to additional benefits, as many of these programs would cut health care costs for the caregivers and beneficiary. (Tilly)
- Measure effectiveness of health care through the reconstitution of social supports and services prior to discharge. (Berman)
- Measure whether patient hospitalizations are noted as observation stays, which make people ineligible for a wide range of services. (Berman)
- Consider a role for CMS in developing a new set of measures that look at population health rather than at individual health. (Berman)
- Develop methods to better define what qualifies as serious illness, perhaps in terms of function and functional limitations, so that practices and systems could better target those individuals who need more than routine care. (Ling)
- Develop quality measures that are appropriate for assessing care of older seriously ill individuals that do not add new reporting burdens on clinicians and that are appropriate for holding providers accountable for serious illness care. (Gosline, Jackson, James, Stevenson, Wang)

**Improving Medicare**

- Establish the ability to have home-based primary care and home-based pre-palliative care reimbursed in Medicare fee-for-service. (Harris)
- Change the prognosis standard for hospice, which is clinically arbitrary and difficult to follow, and eliminate the requirement to forgo disease-modifying therapies. (Debono, Stevenson)
- Ask CMS to consider guidance to allow Medicare hospice providers to offer 24-hour home health aide services to patients at home, rather than requiring them to be transferred to a skilled nursing facility or acute care hospital. (Lee)
- Learn from the lessons hospice has created over the past 30 years, which inform approaches to improve care throughout the health care system. (Banach)
- Develop creative approaches to allow providers to be accountable for drug spending in Medicare. (Harris)

**Expanding Palliative Care**

- Encourage payers, both government and commercial, to reward organizations/providers who demonstrate palliative care competency and quality, if expanded palliative care capacity is desired. (Fine)
- Include incentives in the salary structure for every senior leader in the organization to build these programs. (Fine)
- Develop convincing arguments for palliative care that address issues that leadership finds important. (Jackson)
- Expand efforts to train providers in the principles of palliative care to extend the reach of palliative care. (Popiel)

for potential actions from individual workshop participants. Appendix A contains the workshop Statement of Task and Appendix B contains the workshop agenda. The workshop speakers' presentations have been archived online (as PDF and audio files).[4]

## PATIENT–CAREGIVER–CLINICIAN PERSPECTIVE ON MANAGING AND PAYING FOR SERIOUS ILLNESS CARE

Ralph Bencivenga, a 66-year-old two-time cancer survivor, proud father of three adult children, and caregiver for Patricia, his wife of 45 years who passed away in June 2017, opened the first session by describing the health challenges his wife had faced. Patricia had developed COPD, asthma, emphysema, and cancer. He explained that caring for his wife was difficult. After Patricia became ill, Ralph had to prepare all of their meals, but unlike his wife, he was not a talented cook. He also had to take care of the grocery shopping, banking, laundry, ironing, and yard work, responsibilities that his wife had managed during their many years of marriage. Their home of 25 years had three stories, which made it difficult for Patricia because she could not climb stairs without great effort. Ralph shared that Patricia also needed help with bathing and dressing.

Session moderator Patricia Bomba, vice president and medical director for geriatrics at Excellus BlueCross BlueShield, turned to Bethann Scarborough, associate director of ambulatory services and assistant professor of palliative medicine at the Icahn School of Medicine at Mount Sinai, to get a clearer picture of the specific challenges faced by the couple. Scarborough, who was Ralph and Patricia's palliative care physician for the past few years, explained that Ralph was diagnosed with esophageal cancer in 2012. Ralph received chemotherapy and radiation therapy until his tumor had sufficiently shrunk to be removed surgically. From February 2013 through September 2014, follow-up imaging scans showed no evidence of cancer. Ralph's September 2014 scan, however, identified a lung nodule that was found after a biopsy to be metastatic esophageal cancer. He resumed chemotherapy until March 2015, when additional radiation therapy helped put him into remission. Subsequent imaging scans have not revealed any active disease. However, the chemotherapy significantly exac-

---

[4] For additional information, see http://www.nationalacademies.org/hmd/Activities/HealthServices/QualityCareforSeriousIllnessRoundtable/2017-NOV-29.aspx (accessed January 1, 2018).

erbated Ralph's long-standing, painful peripheral neuropathy in his feet that makes it difficult for him to walk normally, let alone care for someone else.

Meanwhile, Patricia, who had long-standing COPD, had her first contact with Scarborough's hospital in Spring 2016. Tests conducted to investigate nodules present in her lungs found the nodules to be benign, but did reveal a tumor in her colon. A surgical oncologist evaluated her and said the tumor could be surgically removed. However, the surgeon was worried that she would never come off a ventilator because of her COPD, which was so severe that just getting dressed left Patricia breathless, and she was essentially homebound. At that point, Patricia was referred to Scarborough to help facilitate the difficult conversations regarding next steps. "We had a conversation about what was important to her," said Scarborough. "She really did not want to go through with the surgery [and] . . . subsequently decided to enroll in hospice." However, she had second thoughts a few months later and decided to have surgery. The surgery was successful, but over the course of the following year, Patricia had repeated hospital admissions for COPD exacerbations.

At the same time, Scarborough was helping Ralph adjust the pain medications for his peripheral neuropathy, and during their monthly appointments, he would report that Patricia was going back and forth between the hospital and rehabilitation, with short stays at home. Scarborough convinced Ralph to make an appointment for all three of them to talk because it sounded as though managing Patricia's care was becoming increasingly difficult for both Ralph and Patricia. When they failed to keep that appointment, Scarborough called Ralph, who told her that his wife was too sick to leave the house. At that point, Scarborough arranged for home hospice, but Patricia died that same day.

When Bomba asked Ralph to describe his experience caring for his wife, he started by describing her as a very shy yet proud and independent woman. As Patricia's illness progressed and she became less and less able to perform normal activities, "She would just sit there and cry," Ralph recalled. He described how he needed to both do the cooking and feed his wife because she was unable to coordinate her movements by that point. Ralph compared that experience to caring for a seventh grandchild. He also noted the difficulty he was having navigating the stairs in his three-story house and said that it was only with Scarborough's help managing his pain medications that he was able to keep going. Scarborough added that doing so was challenging given the need to balance pain control and Ralph's need to be functional enough to care for his wife. Compounding the challenge of counseling the couple was the fact that Patricia was often going to other hospitals, which made it hard for Scarborough to track the progression of her illness.

Turning to the subject of how his and Patricia's illnesses affected their finances, Ralph said that during the 35 years he worked as an executive for Merrill Lynch, the company provided health insurance covered nearly all of the hospital bills, and his annual performance bonuses took care of the non-covered costs. When he lost his job, he lost his coverage and enrolled in a Consolidated Omnibus Budget Reconciliation Act (COBRA) plan,[5] which cost him between $1,600 and $2,000 per month and he likened to having an additional mortgage. The cost of insurance and co-payments for every hospital stay kept adding up, eventually totaling approximately $110,000, which he had to withdraw from his retirement savings. In addition, he received a $30,000 bill for the 40 days his wife spent in a rehabilitation center that his health plan would not cover. Ralph had been hospitalized at the time and had failed to get preauthorization for her stay.

Scarborough noted that the monthly cost of Ralph's medications was running close to $2,000. Further compounding the situation, the Bencivengas did not have coverage for home health care. "Without that, there was no ability to get somebody into the home to help with things without having to have the family privately hire someone, which is expensive and just not possible for many families," said Scarborough.

When Bomba asked Ralph if the hospital offered any support for him and Patricia, he explained that he was given the number of a social worker, who helped to arrange for a visiting nurse to come to the house for 3 to 4 hours per week to help care for Patricia. That care, however, involved little more than sitting with Patricia and watching television, Ralph explained, whereas the Bencivengas needed help with daily activities such as household chores and cooking. Ralph noted that hiring a private health aide would have been prohibitively expensive. He also explained that one of his biggest challenges was getting Patricia from their home on Staten Island to her appointments at Mount Sinai, given that she was no longer ambulatory.

---

[5] COBRA gives workers and their families who lose their health benefits the right to choose to continue group health benefits provided by their group health plan for limited periods of time at their own expense under certain circumstances such as voluntary or involuntary job loss, reduction in the hours worked, transition between jobs, death, divorce, and other life events. For more information, see https://www.dol.gov/general/topic/health-plans/cobra (accessed February 23, 2018).

One-way taxi fare was more than $100, while taking the subway required walking much longer distances than Patricia could manage.

In Ralph and Patricia's case, home health visits would have been enormously helpful, but as Scarborough pointed out, figuring out how to pay for them was the challenge. "We do not currently have that kind of infrastructure in place to be able to do that," she said. At one point, she added, Ralph's condition had stabilized to the point where he could work with his local primary physician to adjust his medication, rather than having to visit Scarborough to do so. However, over the past year, his condition was not stable enough to allow that.

When asked if he signed up for Meals on Wheels, Ralph replied he did, but his wife was such a picky eater that she would not eat the food provided by the program or similar programs. Bomba asked Ralph if Patricia's physicians had let him know that her appetite might not be normal given how ill she was, and Ralph replied that Patricia's physicians never talked to him about what to expect as her health continued to deteriorate. "I have to tell you, I thought I would have her for another couple of years," said Ralph. He added that if he had known what little time Patricia had left, he would have exhausted his funds to give her a better quality of life for the last few weeks when she was dying at home or put her into hospice sooner—which Scarborough had recommended.

Ralph currently has about half of his retirement funds remaining and owes approximately $150,000 on a home equity loan he took out to pay for his and Patricia's medical expenses. He has taken a job to keep himself busy and help cover his expenses. Bomba asked if he ever thought of declaring bankruptcy, and he said no, pointing out proudly that he has paid all his bills on time for the past 48 years.

Scarborough described how she felt helpless as a clinician, knowing there were things that both Ralph and Patricia needed as patients and in Ralph's role as caregiver, but she did not have a way to provide them. She explained, "We have pills to fix a lot of things, but we do not have a pill for caregiving and for help with the day-to-day things that can help control symptoms at home, reduce caregiver burden, and help keep people out of the hospital if the hospital is not where they want to be or where they need to be if the medical care can be provided in the home." Scarborough added, "I think it is really challenging to have the kind of health infrastructure that we have in this country and still see all the enumerable places where people fall through the cracks because no one is helping people outside of the hospital setting." Bomba agreed that the current financing and payment system is focused on hospitalizations and medications, but what Patricia wanted most was to be cared for in her own home.

Bomba closed the discussion by thanking Ralph for sharing his experience, and noted that his story helped shine a light on the difficult reality of health care financing for many Americans, as well as the magnitude of caregiver needs. In thinking about the nation's aging population and the fact that so many older Americans have needs similar to those of the Bencivengas, Bomba said, "We need to be able to move from focusing on purely the medical needs to addressing a lot of these very basic human needs to be able to allow folks to stay in their home." As a final thought, she shared that she appreciated Ralph's love for Patricia and what he was able to accomplish in what were very difficult circumstances.

## FRAMING THE CHALLENGES AND OPPORTUNITES FOR FINANCING AND PAYMENT INNOVATION

David Stevenson, associate professor of health policy at Vanderbilt University School of Medicine, began his presentation by pointing out that financing approaches are integral components of serious illness and end-of-life care. Financing approaches influence both access and quality of care, as well as costs, and determine how services will be paid. In providing context on why these issues are so important, Stevenson noted that policy discussions tend to focus on the cost of serious illness and end-of-life care. Stevenson explained that although many people who are at the end of life do have high health care costs, it is important to understand that approximately 90 percent of the high-cost population is not at the end of life (Aldridge and Kelley, 2015). Most individuals with high health care costs are those with serious illnesses, particularly chronic illnesses such as cancer, emphysema, COPD, and Alzheimer's disease and other forms of dementia, as well as the range of functional limitations that often accompany those conditions. Furthermore, most people with serious illness live with their conditions for a long time, which is why long-term services and supports and caregiving are so critical for this population. "It is not just care at the end of life," Stevenson emphasized.

Given that the large share of individuals with serious illness are more than 65 years old, Medicare plays a substantial role in shaping serious illness care in the United States through its coverage of a range of inpatient, outpatient, post-acute home health services, skilled nurse facility care, and so on, said Stevenson. Medicare's hospice benefit, the primary mechanism for financing end-of-life care, encompasses a broad array of palliative and support services, but is limited to individuals with a terminal diagnosis who are willing to forgo curative therapies. Stevenson pointed out the substantial gaps between coverage and need—particularly for things such as long-term services and supports, transportation, and nutritional services that can benefit an individual more than another hospitalization—as well as high cost sharing and limited coverage for palliative care outside of hospice. "If you are thinking about outpatient palliative care, meeting people where they are in the community, there is very limited coverage of that in the Medicare program," said Stevenson.

Stevenson explained that approximately 80 percent of people who die each year are Medicare beneficiaries (Aldridge and Kelley, 2015), so "what Medicare does in terms of its end-of-life care really matters a great deal," he explained. He noted that a common misconception is that end-of-life care accounts for an increasing share of the Medicare budget, when in fact the share of program spending for people at the end of their lives has been relatively steady at approximately 25 percent (Cubanski et al., 2016). What has changed, though, is the care people receive at the end of life, with an increase in the role of hospice care. Despite this increased role, approximately two-thirds of Medicare beneficiaries are hospitalized in the last month of their lives, often spending time in the intensive care unit. Stevenson added that many of the same challenges affecting end-of-life care, such as siloed financing and fragmented service delivery, also affect serious illness care (Teno et al., 2013).

Stevenson further explained that Medicare's influence extends beyond those it covers directly, given that Medicaid and private insurers "often follow Medicare's lead in some good ways and not so good ways," explained Stevenson. Some commercial plans, for example, are exploring alternative approaches, including financing earlier use of palliative care and a broader conception of the hospice benefit. As with Medicare, most commercial plans do not cover long-term services and supports, though some are experimenting with providing targeted social supports. While hospice and palliative care are not included in the 10 essential benefits of the Patient Protection and Affordable Care Act of 2010 (ACA) plans, every state's benchmark plans do include those benefits (HHS, 2013). Stevenson noted that the increasing use of high-deductible health plans in recent years amplifies the financial burden on patients and families.

Stevenson noted that individuals with serious illness typically have high out-of-pocket costs arising from coverage gaps. Referring to the six-figure out-of-pocket costs Ralph and Patricia accrued, Stevenson emphasized that most people do not have the resources to bear those costs. One study, for example, found that average out-of-pocket costs—not total health care spending—were nearly $40,000 over the last 5 years of life (see Figure 1). Nursing home care accounts for a large portion of those out-of-pocket expenses, even though most people in nursing homes are there because they need assistance with daily life activities and not necessarily traditional medical care, Stevenson explained. He added that prescription drug costs can also account for a substantial share of an individual's out-of-pocket costs even when the individual is covered by insurance (Kelley et al., 2013).

One of Medicare's design flaws, Stevenson noted, is its siloed approach to what services individuals are eligible for, the extent of that

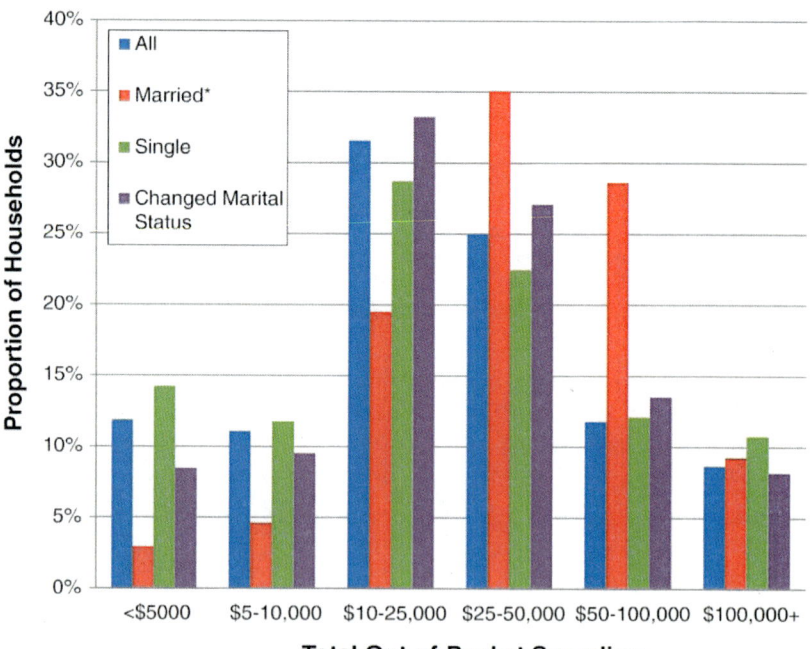

**FIGURE 1** Distribution of out-of-pocket spending in the last 5 years of life.
* Expenditures for married include expenses of both spouse and household head.
SOURCES: As presented by David Stevenson, November 29, 2017; Kelley et al., 2013.

coverage, and how it pays for those benefits. Medicare pays for inpatient benefits separately from outpatient benefits, post-acute rehabilitative care, end-of-life care, home health care, and skilled nursing facility (SNF) care. Patients, families, and their medical providers often struggle with this piecemeal approach, Stevenson noted, adding, "the fee-for-service part of Medicare really does not incentivize strong coordination of care across settings and benefits."

Although hospice care is the primary federally financed mechanism for end-of-life care, the eligibility policy serves to limit the use of this benefit. These eligibility provisions, Stevenson explained, were designed to limit the cost of the benefit. Nonetheless, hospice use has grown substantially over its 30-plus year history and today, approximately half of Medicare recipients use the benefit before they die and 35 percent of those who use the benefit are in nursing homes and assisted living facilities (Gozalo et al., 2015). Referring to hospice as "this great escape hatch in some ways from the fee-for-service systems that push people toward more and higher intensity use," Stevenson noted, however, that hospice is not relevant to the 90 percent of high-cost patients who are not at the end of life.

What is needed, Stevenson asserted, is a more integrated approach to caring for people with serious illness that addresses their interconnected needs, whether those are physical, psychological, supportive, and/or spiritual. "In the context of policy, we do not think that way typically," said Stevenson, but as the IOM's 2015 *Dying in America* report noted, piecemeal reforms will not be effective. "We need to think much more comprehensively about a different mix of medical and social services than are currently brought to bear for individuals with serious illness," he said, adding that financing and payment reform should prioritize benefits such as caregiver training and support, home modifications, meals and nutrition, and transportation over some of the medical benefits now provided. One important caveat, also noted in *Dying in America*, is that increasing spending and benefits without other value-based reforms is not feasible in the current political context (IOM, 2015). Stevenson framed the question of value "in terms of whether it is earlier access to palliative care or other supportive services, preventing hospitalizations, reducing complications that can arise," as an important test to pass.

Stevenson noted that efforts are under way to experiment with innovative, value-based financing and delivery strategies that aim to rationalize and improve care for people with serious illness. These include primary care and care management models, bundled payment demonstrations, accountable care organizations (ACOs),[6] and various managed care approaches such as Medicare Advantage, special needs plans (SNPs),[7] and patient-centered medical homes.[8] Stevenson emphasized that "financial incentives need to be aligned with accountability to ensure that these value-based approaches do not result in diminished quality of care."

Stevenson emphasized the importance of including palliative care and hospice in these models to the extent feasible. In many models, such as those that bundle payments, patients enrolling in hospice are removed from the demonstration, explained Stevenson. The same is true with the financial alignment demonstrations for individuals eligible for both Medicare and Medicaid. "We need to think more holistically about these programs to really impact the whole of the person who has a serious illness," he said.

To conclude his presentation, Stevenson identified four key financing challenges. First, he explained that "Medicare and other types of insurance . . . do not cover all services that people [with serious illness] need." He noted lack of coverage for long-term services and supports is the most prominent problem, but other needs can pose a substantial burden on a patient's finances. While Medicaid provides a "limited safety net . . . it is not sufficient for [many individuals with serious illness]." This results in substantial out-of-pocket costs, especially for those living with serious illness over an extended period. Furthermore, Stevenson asserts that the scrutiny placed on ensuring that hospice and home health benefits do not become

---

[6] ACOs are groups of doctors, hospitals, and other health care providers who come together voluntarily to provide coordinated care to their Medicare patients. Medicare ACOs include Shared Savings Program, Advance Payment ACO, and Pioneer ACO. For more information, see https://www.cms.gov/Medicare/Medicare-Fee-for-Service-Payment/ACO (accessed February 23, 2018). See also https://khn.org/news/aco-accountable-care-organization-faq (accessed February 23, 2018).

[7] Medicare SNPs are a type of Medicare Advantage Plan that limits membership to people with specific diseases or characteristics. SNPs tailor their benefits, provider choices, and drug formularies to the specific needs of the groups they serve. For more information, see https://www.medicare.gov/sign-up-change-plans/medicare-health-plans/medicare-advantage-plans/special-needs-plans.html (accessed February 23, 2018).

[8] The patient-centered medical home is a model of care where patients have a direct relationship with a provider who coordinates a cooperative team of health care professionals that take collective responsibility for the integrated care provided to the patient. The team can also advocate and arrange care for the patient with other qualified providers and community resources. For more information, see https://pcmh.ahrq.gov/page/defining-pcmh (accessed February 23, 2018).

a de facto long-term care benefit can take the focus away from providing high-quality care.

The second financing challenge that Stevenson identified relates to hospice eligibility. Stevenson explained that the 6-month "prognosis standard is clinically arbitrary and difficult to follow, particularly for [patients] with non-cancer diagnoses," and the requirement to forgo disease-modifying therapies enforces an artificial distinction and impedes timely enrollment, resulting in very short hospice stays. About 25 percent of hospice stays are 5 days or less (MedPAC, 2017), which is not enough time to provide much benefit for those individuals. He emphasized that access to palliative care is often limited in the community setting.

The third challenge is that with the exception of ACOs, hospice is generally excluded from integrated financing and delivery demonstrations systems such as Bundled Payments for Care Improvement (BPCI)[9] or Programs of All-Inclusive Care for the Elderly (PACE).[10] Medicare Advantage plans, for example, drop enrollees in hospice except for provision of supplemental services. Although this "carve out" ensures access to an individual's hospice provider of choice, it reduces the incentives for Medicare Advantage plans to bolster their own expertise and creates incentives for plans to cede responsibility for end-of-life care.

The fourth financing challenge highlighted by Stevenson arises from the fact that as the health care system increasingly focuses on value, there are few established quality measures to hold providers accountable for serious illness care. Currently, none of the 33 performance measures included in the ACA relate to end-of-life care,[11] and as a result, said Stevenson, providers and plans are not always attuned to providing high-quality palliative and end-of-life care.

---

[9] BPCI was created by the Center for Medicare & Medicaid Innovation (CMMI) to test four different models of care that involve an inpatient hospital stay in order to incentivize providers to better coordinate care by paying for related care as part of a broad payment bundle and treat a patient during a single episode. For more information, see https://innovation.cms.gov/initiatives/bpci-advanced (accessed February 23, 2018).

[10] PACE is a Medicare and Medicaid program designed to allow people to receive health care in the community rather than staying in a nursing home or care facility. For more information, see https://www.medicare.gov/your-medicare-costs/help-paying-costs/pace/pace.html (accessed February 23, 2018).

[11] For more information, see https://www.cms.gov/Medicare/Medicare-Fee-for-Service-Payment/sharedsavingsprogram/Downloads/ACO-Shared-Savings-Program-Quality-Measures.pdf (accessed March 7, 2018).

Though Medicare plays a key role in financing serious illness care in the United States, it has significant coverage gaps and limitations, noted Stevenson. The transition to value-based payment and care delivery represents an opportunity for palliative care and hospice, but progress will be limited if these services are excluded or deemphasized. Stevenson concluded his remarks by noting that in the context of the heightened focus on value and efforts to develop incentives for a more comprehensive approach to providing care for people with serious illness, "it is important not only to have financial incentives that push in that direction, but also accountability standards to make sure providers are delivering" high-quality care.

### Taking Care of a Seriously Ill Patient in the Context of the Current Health Care Financing System

Diane Meier, director of the Center to Advance Palliative Care, agreed with Scarborough's earlier comment on how, when faced with the inability to help patients get the care they need because of gaps in the current system, a clinician can be led to feel like a failure. Meier believes that dealing with this challenge is one of the reasons for the high rate of burnout among physicians today. Meier noted that most large U.S. hospitals now provide palliative care and hospice, and that access to hospice in the United States is the highest for any developed nation (Dumanovsky et al., 2016; The Economist Intelligence Unit, 2015), but as Stevenson pointed out, the vast majority of people with serious illness are not dying and are not eligible for hospice.

To illustrate what caring for a person with serious illness is like, Meier discussed a hypothetical case her organization has developed for an online course on caring for someone with dementia. The main actors in this case are Martha, who in addition to having dementia is frail and suffers from severe and disabling back pain resulting from spinal stenosis and arthritis; Bernard, her husband and primary caregiver; and Dr. Jones, Martha's primary care physician. Early one morning, Martha falls in the bathroom, and a frantic Bernard debates what to do. The doctor's office is closed, so Bernard calls 911. An ambulance service, which may not be in their Medicare plan's network, arrives and takes Martha to the emergency department. After spending the morning there, Martha is admitted for treatment of fecal impaction.

After Martha is discharged, Bernard visits Dr. Jones at his office, where he relays that her agitation has not improved since starting on a laxative and that she lays awake most nights moaning and crying. Bernard adds that he is so exhausted that he has forgotten to give Martha her medicine several times, and Dr. Jones's staff begins to worry about both Bernard and Martha. After determining that Martha cannot participate in a conversation about what is important to her, Dr. Jones talks to Bernard about what he thinks she would want. Martha is terrified of going to a nursing home, says Bernard, and she made him promise to keep her home with him.

Not only is Bernard at his wits' end, but so is Dr. Jones, who has sent home care to their home, only to have Martha discharged from care after a few weeks because she does not have a skilled need, which is required for home health care and is defined as health care that requires a skilled nursing or rehabilitation staff for the purposes of managing, observing, and evaluating care (CMS, 2017b). She is not eligible for hospice, and so she gets episodic care from a certified home health agency, shuttling back and forth between home and hospital. With no alternatives, Dr. Jones believes he is failing his patient until he remembers seeing an email about a house calls program for complex patients in the new Medicare ACO to which his health system belongs. With one phone call, he arranges for home-based primary and palliative care for Martha with a house calls practice in her community. The house calls team visits several times per week until Martha's condition stabilizes. They tell Dr. Jones about the situation the couple faces—no food in the refrigerator, no grab bars or elevated toilet seat in the bathroom, loose rugs and electrical wires everywhere, laundry strewn about—problems that Dr. Jones was not aware of because he had not been in their home.

Now that Dr. Jones knows about the problems, his office arranges for a home health agency to conduct a safety evaluation, install grab bars and an elevated toilet, provide a hospital bed and a chair that assist in standing, and arranges for Meals on Wheels. With Bernard and Martha's permission, the house calls team contacts their church and arranges for a friendly visitor program, something most faith communities provide, and for someone to bring them to church and back home on Sundays. The friendly visitors also allow Bernard to get out to shop and see his friends, which improves his quality of life. Dr. Jones also talks to a palliative care colleague on the house calls team, who reassures him that he can safely prescribe small amounts of morphine to alleviate Martha's back pain along with a laxative for constipation.

When Dr. Jones next sees Bernard, he has gained some weight and no longer appears drawn and depressed. Bernard tells Dr. Jones that both he and Martha are now sleeping through the night, and relays that the occupational therapist from the home health agency downloaded some Broadway show tunes, Martha's favorite music, onto an iPod for her and that she sings along with great gusto. Bernard says he is happy to see Martha take pleasure in life again and that he has his wife back. Better yet, over the next 18 months, Bernard does not have to call 911 or take Martha to the emergency department. Eventually, though, she begins to refuse food and fluids and choke on her food, and Dr. Jones considers a hospice referral so that Martha can continue to remain comfortable at home.

To Meier, this case study represents the promise of home-based primary and palliative care. Before Dr. Jones remembered the email notice about ACO coverage for home-based care, there were four 911 calls in a 3-month period leading to four emergency department visits and three hospitalizations, which in turn led to a hospital-acquired infection, functional decline for Martha, and family distress. "The system is perfectly designed to get the results it gets," Meier said. After calling the house calls team, Martha's pain was better managed, Bernard had 24/7 phone coverage and support, and Meals on Wheels and his faith community provided support. There were no 911 calls, emergency department visits, or hospitalizations, and Martha passed away peacefully at home after receiving 5 months of hospice care.

What made it possible to provide more appropriate and better care for Martha and Bernard was a value-based payment model enabled by a risk-bearing entity, which in this case was a Medicare ACO, explained Meier. She noted that most home-based palliative care programs are sponsored by an ACO such as ProHEALTH's practice-based ACO and Sharp HealthCare's pioneer ACO (ProHEALTH, 2017; Sharp HealthCare, 2017). In closing, she stressed that "When you have financial alignment with the right care, it can make a huge difference in meeting patients' needs."

## Discussion

During the discussion session following the presentations, Bomba asked about cost avoidance analysis. Meier responded that studies show substantial cost avoidance from these types of value-based models. Sean Morrison, director of the National Palliative Care Research Center at Mount Sinai, pointed to a potential problem with value-based care and cost avoidance. He noted that while formal health care costs might decline, there could be a shift of cost onto patients and families, who then have to secure community-based services for which they may have to pay. He cited an experience in Edmonton, Canada, where enhancing palliative care options in the community did reduce formal health care costs but shifted costs onto patients and families. "I think we need to keep that in mind as we promote value-based care," he said, adding that studies are needed that look beyond direct health care costs and examine the informal costs of care and patient and family outcomes. Morrison asked the speakers if there are payment sources that would meet the needs of someone like Ralph. Stevenson responded that much of the initial work in terms of what ACOs are doing has focused on the post-acute side given the scope of variation in spending. He agreed with Morrison that information on the impact on families is currently not available and quantitative studies are necessary.

Shari Ling from CMS, referring to the challenge of trying to provide integrated services through individual programs and benefits tied to specific authorities, asked everyone to think about what could be accomplished "in the here and now" through guidance that may provide alternative interpretations of current statutes. To that point, Bomba inquired whether that might include guidance to ACOs that shared savings might encompass, for example, a voucher program that caregivers could use for their individual needs. Ling responded that it would depend on the program, but "there are so many nuances, it is worth thinking about what would be most helpful." Ling added that CMS has made progress in identifying caregiver needs as part of some assessments. She stressed the importance of looking at each program and learning about what might be most helpful in terms of saving costs and improving outcomes. Workshop participant Jane Tilly from the Administration for Community Living suggested that the unit for cost analysis related to additional benefits might be beneficiary and caregiver costs combined. She said she suspects strongly that many of these programs would cut health care costs for caregivers as well as the beneficiary.

Amy Berman from The John A. Hartford Foundation, responding to Ling's challenge to identify changes, which are "low-hanging fruit" that can be accomplished through interpretation versus changing the statute, wondered about "balanced measures" and whether measuring factors such as reconstitution of social supports and services prior to discharge might be one way to measure effectiveness. She said there is much discussion about whether patient hospitalizations are treated as observation stays, which render people ineligible for a range of services. She asked about CMS's role in interpreting a new set of measures that look at population health.

Berman also asked about potential changes to the unit of care. Recognizing the complexities of family caregiving, and how a person's ability to receive care at home depends on the support of the caregiver, Berman wondered if it is within CMS's purview to include the family as the unit of care, given the precedent to do so for disability care within Medicare. "Maybe it is simply taking the current interpretation and thinking about this in ways that broaden the interpretation to a changing society," suggested Berman.

Teresa Lee from VNA Health Group suggested that one place where CMS guidance might help would be in the area of home hospice. She noted that in order for patients and caregivers to take advantage of the respite benefit in hospice, the patient has to be transferred to an SNF or acute care hospital. She wondered if CMS might consider allowing Medicare hospice providers to offer 24-hour home health aide services to patients at home.

Thinking back to Morrison's and Stevenson's comments, Ling wondered if there are sources for the type of cost data they seek, she said. "It may be beyond CMS authority to receive those data," and yet the data may be available elsewhere. Meier pointed out that some government-supported surveys, such as the Health and Retirement Survey,[12] do measure the effect of health care on individual and family finances. Stevenson commented that giving researchers broader access to Medicare Advantage encounter data might provide answers to some important questions on value and cost. He pointed out that one-third of Medicare beneficiaries enroll in Medicare Advantage programs, and Medicare Advantage beneficiaries enroll in hospice in greater numbers than in traditional Medicare programs (Jacobson et al., 2017). However, little is known about the care they receive before enrolling in hospice or what kind of care they get if they do not enroll in hospice.

Kelly Vontran, who works at CMS on payment policy for home health and hospice, said that getting data from providers on the impact of social determinants of health on how and if patients access health care can be challenging, and it is difficult to determine whether the information is accurate and not "just an artifact of a payment incentive." She asked about effective ways to get critical information about social determinants of health, for example, so that high-quality comprehensive care can be provided to patients with serious illness.

Judith Peres from the Social Work Hospice and Palliative Care Network asked the panelists for their thoughts on how it might be possible to coordinate services provided by the health system with the types of

---

[12] The Health and Retirement Survey is a longitudinal project sponsored by the National Institute on Aging and the Social Security Administration and was conducted at the University of Michigan's Institute for Social Research. For more information, see http://hrsonline.isr.umich.edu (accessed March 5, 2018).

services offered through Independence at Home, including transportation, food and nutrition, and home modifications (NASEM, 2017c). Stevenson emphasized that it is counterproductive to divide people's needs into acute, post-acute, end-of-life, and long-term services and supports, given that they are all connected. His hope is that the U.S. Senate's eventual passage of the CHRONIC Care Act,[13] which extends the Independence at Home demonstration program and expands supplemental benefits to meet the needs of chronically ill Medicare Advantage enrollees, will lead to more experimentation and more awareness among physicians so that they can try to secure non-medical services to address their patients' needs.

Jeanne Chirico, vice president for community services for Lifetime Care and director of the Excellus BlueCross BlueShield CompassionNet program, commented that one problem with huge funding streams, such as those that finance ACOs, is that they take resources away from community-based organizations. To her, the challenge is to develop a network of community-based organizations that receive funds directly to provide needed services instead of having funds trickle down from the acute care system. She said that CMS has approved one social ACO and would like to see more work in this area.[14]

## EXPLORING FINANCING AND PAYMENT INNOVATIONS: CHALLENGES, IMPACTS, AND LESSONS FROM FEE-FOR-SERVICE AND VALUE-BASED PAYMENT ARRANGEMENTS

In his introduction to the workshop's second session, Harold Paz, executive vice president and chief medical officer at Aetna, explained that quality care for people with serious illness is a high-priority area for Aetna and is the focus of its Compassionate Care program. This program identifies Aetna members with serious illness, coordinates their care, and provides

---

[13] The Creating High-Quality Results and Outcomes Necessary to Improve Chronic Care Act (CHRONIC) improves the Medicare program by focusing on traditional fee-for-service, Medicare Advantage, and ACOs and expands the Independence at Home demonstration program. For more information, see https://www.congress.gov/bill/115th-congress/senate-bill/870 (accessed March 5, 2018) and https://www.finance.senate.gov/imo/media/doc/CHRONIC%20Care%20Act%20of%202017%20One-Pager%204.6.17.pdf (accessed March 5, 2018).

[14] Social ACOs serve populations with complex and unmet social and economic needs that impact health outcomes, such as housing, food security, and employment. See https://www.healthaffairs.org/do/10.1377/hblog20170125.058419/full (accessed March 5, 2018).

counseling to improve quality of life and support end-of-life preferences. When the company launched the program more a decade ago, it decided to offer both palliative care and hospice care for a full year instead of 6 months, and to cover it concurrently with acute care services so that a member would not have to choose between the two.

Paz noted that Aetna's data showed that members in the program had significantly lower usage of acute care services, including hospitalization in the intensive care unit, emergency department visits, and medical–surgical procedures. According to internal data, members in the program also reported high levels of patient satisfaction to go along with more than $12,000 in lower expenditures on average during the last year of life. Subsequent analysis of data from a matched control study showed significant reductions in emergency department visits and inpatient acute admission, as well as a 13 percent reduction in total medical costs, according to Paz. Moreover, Compassionate Care program beneficiaries were also 36 percent more likely to use hospice and had an average stay in hospice that was 37 percent longer than for the control group.[15] In Paz's view, this program is a model of how payers can provide managed care services that offer superior value for patients. "As we move toward patient-centered personalized health, care management—along with interoperability of patient-centered data and information and value-based contracting—offers the opportunity to create a new way of delivering services for individuals at the end of life, and frankly, I think, across the entire life span," said Paz.

**Financing Serious Illness Care at Cambia Health Solutions**

For Cambia Health Solutions, creating a personalized health care solution for every person under their care is a cause, not a mission, said Richard Popiel, Cambia's executive vice president and chief medical officer. He pointed out that the best example of the commitment to that cause is how Cambia addresses palliative and end-of-life care. The organization established Cambia Health Foundation in 2007 as its vehicle for funding its work on palliative care. In 2009, the foundation funded the University of Washington's hospital-based palliative care center, now known as the Cambia Palliative Care Center of Excellence. Popiel shared anecdotal evidence that the center is starting to realize the anticipated returns and outcomes.

In addition, Popiel noted that the foundation has funded an endowed

---

[15] Information was unpublished/in press at the time of this proceedings' publication.

chair for pediatric palliative care at the Oregon Health & Science University. It also funds the Sojourns Scholar Leadership Program, which trains 10 clinicians—physicians, nurses, social workers, physician assistants, chaplains, psychologists, pharmacists, and other emerging health system leaders—with the goal of creating the next generation of palliative care leaders. The program is in its fourth year and has trained 40 individuals.

The Cambia Health Foundation has also partnered with Blue Cross Blue Shield of North Carolina (BCBSNC) in Echo Health Ventures, which invests in companies aligned with its cause. One such company, GNS HealthCare, which works in artificial intelligence and machine learning, has developed an algorithm that identifies patients likely to die within the next 12 months. Popiel said that Cambia Health Solutions is using this algorithm to identify members who would likely benefit from palliative care case management services. These are examples, according to Popiel, of "how we have leaned in financially and committed to addressing some of the gaps that exist in palliative care."

Turning to work that Cambia has been involved in with its regional health plans, Popiel explained that in 2012–2013, Cambia Health Solutions initiated a benchmarking exercise, which involved speaking with palliative care experts, consumers, and providers, to identify what it could be doing as a health plan to serve its members more effectively needing palliative and end-of-life care. This information enabled Cambia to perform a gap analysis, which subsequently led to a sweeping change in the benefits the company offered. It also led to the creation of a specialized case management program that includes caregiver support, regardless of whether the caregiver is a plan member. Cambia also inventoried all services available in the communities it serves. Its case managers use that inventory to help members navigate the range of available services in their communities. In addition to providing caregiver support, Cambia's health benefit plan for serious illness care now includes advance care planning—with no limits on the number of discussions between the patient and the provider. Cambia also funds home health medical and psychosocial services and, recognizing that "providers who have been caring for their patients for a long time also grieve," Cambia provides support for health care providers as well. The plan does not require Medicare Advantage members to be homebound to access these services, nor does it require prior authorization for therapies. These services are available for members of any age and for any diagnosis.

In closing, Popiel noted that Cambia is continually evaluating how best to serve seriously ill patients and their program is dynamic. Although financial impact is always a consideration, funding determinations are driven by "what is best for our members. We want to personalize the situation for them," said Popiel.

**CompassionNet: Community-Based Pediatric Palliative Care**

Jeanne Chirico, vice president for community services for Lifetime Care and director of the Excellus BlueCross BlueShield CompassionNet program, explained that CompassionNet is a community-based pediatric palliative care program covering some 300 square miles in upstate New York, including low-income rural areas as well as urban centers such as Buffalo, Rochester, and Syracuse. As a wrap-around program, it supports the entire family as a unit and provides for all of their needs—psychosocial, financial, medical, or environmental. The program's services are offered to every child who a physician believes is at significant risk of dying before age 21. Children with an acute exacerbation of a chronic illness that increases their risk of dying before adulthood also are eligible for the program.

Chirico explained that CompassionNet was created when Lifetime Care heard from its families that it was not doing a good job caring for their seriously ill children. At the same time, Excellus, which owns Lifetime Care, learned that it was doing a poor job as well, for instance, by issuing denial letters in the mail for services that these children needed. In an effort to address this situation, Excellus allowed Lifetime Care to develop a program that does not replicate any service that is already in the community or any service that is not needed. "This is not a want program, it is a need program," explained Chirico. The primary goal of the program is to provide qualified staff, education, and emotional support to families and allow for a realistic option for their child to die at home should that become necessary, said Chirico, though she noted that approximately 30 percent of the children in the program go into remission or are cured.

Lifetime Care built collaborations with hundreds of community-based organizations, forming a network of services available to any family member. After a licensed social worker completes a needs assessment with the child and family to determine their biggest stressor, they arrange for services to address those needs. Services may include expressive therapies such as art, music, and dance/movement, for example, for the child who is ill, and/or their siblings who may not understand what is happening. Massage therapy may also be provided for the child and mother who is caring for her child non-stop. In other instances, assistance with finances may be provided to families facing financial hardship that results from caring for a seriously ill child. As an example of the latter, Chirico explained that a family might be faced with having their utilities turned off because they had spent all their money on medical bills. Case managers will go to community resources and find funds to help with that issue and put a plan in place to ensure it does not happen again. She noted that the cost of providing these services has not been exorbitant.

While the goal of this program is to comfort families and provide them with the realistic option of having their child die at home, it is not designed to replace hospice, but to provide specialized expertise for programs that may not be experienced in pediatric palliative care services for children at the end of life. In addition, this program has produced cost savings for the payer and high parental satisfaction, Chirico said.

Citing data from the National Hospice and Palliative Care Organization, Chirico pointed out that fewer than 20 percent of children with serious illness die at home (CMS, 2017c) (see Figure 2). By contrast, more than half of the children ages 1 to 19 participating in CompassionNet died at home, with those dying in the hospital being largely the result of parental preference, such as when parents do not want their other children to witness their sibling's death. Chirico pointed out the importance of this issue, noting, "This is about quality." She added "studies have shown that when families can make that decision about where they want this event to occur, their bereavement is better, and their health is better" (IOM, 2003).

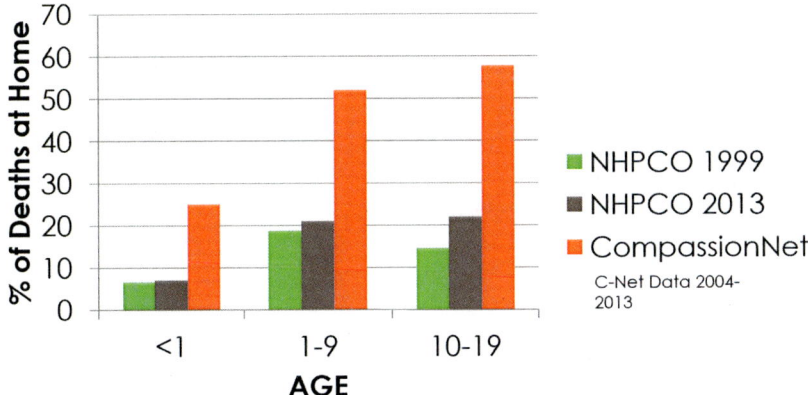

**FIGURE 2** Deaths at home by age.
NOTE: NHPCO = National Hospice and Palliative Care Organization.
SOURCES: As presented by Jeanne Chirico, November 29, 2017; CMS, 2017c.

Chirico referred to a recent internal cost analysis using claims data for all of the children who died between 2008 and 2015 (see Table 1). The analysis revealed that helping families get the support they need to feel safe at home and have their child die at home produces enough cost-of-care savings to pay for the entire program for every child. "This is a shift of expense that improves outcomes, quality of care, bereavement support, and the health and well-being of siblings and parents," said Chirico. On a final note, she added that when thinking about community-based organizations, there is a method and a systematic way to bring communities together in a way to ensure these types of results.

### Anthem's Enhanced Personal Health Care

When the leadership at Anthem studied how its members with serious illness were receiving care, they found fragmented care between primary care providers and specialists characterized by limited advance care planning, inadequate symptom control, aggressive care near the end of life (including in-patient hospitalizations and chemotherapy), and limited hospice usage. In response, said David Debono, medical director for oncology at Anthem, Inc., the organization developed its Enhanced Personal Health Care program, a value-based payment program involving more than 50,000 providers and caring for more than 4.5 million members with a clinical goal of improving patient-centered care. The palliative care piece of this program works to identify high-risk members with daily hot-spotter reports that enable the company to shift resources to serve these members better. The program also relies on monthly data feeds to identify care gaps and risk stratify members on a regular basis.

For providers to participate in this program, they must agree to provide members with 24/7 access through extended office hours and after-hours call coverage, and they must have a dedicated position within their practice to support participation in the program. Debono explained that providers and staff, who regularly participate in collaborative learning sessions, learn to use a disease registry to manage patients with chronic conditions. In addition, they must be willing to engage in care planning for high-risk populations and in quality and performance measurement.

Debono explained that there is a significant upfront investment—particularly in terms of human resources—for practices that join the program. Transformation teams from Anthem help practices transition from a fee-for-service model to a value-based model, and a clinical liaison works

**TABLE 1** Cost and Location of Death at Five Moments in the Last Year of Life

| | Median Total Costs | | | | |
|---|---|---|---|---|---|
| | Year | 6 Months | 3 Months | 1 Month | Last Week |
| Children/Adolescents | | | | | |
| Hospital (n = 84) | $197,069 | $113,110 | $67,561 | $45,615 | $29,169 |
| Home (n = 74) | $116,708 | $57,295 | $24,521 | $6,173 | $1,213 |
| Mann-Whitney U (p) | 2,269 (.003) | 2,013 (<.001) | 1,648 (<.001) | 1,149 (<.001) | 729 (<.001) |
| Infants | | | | | |
| Hospital (n = 51) | $111,876 | $111,876 | $111,876 | $94,025 | $78,442 |
| Home (n = 14) | $94,009 | $77,406 | $23,375 | $12,508 | $2,288 |
| Mann-Whitney U (p) | 302 (.38) | 240 (.06) | 137 (<.001) | 86 (<.001) | 65 (<.001) |

NOTE: P values are based on two-tailed tests.
SOURCE: Adapted from Chirico presentation, November 29, 2017; based on internal actuarial data.

regularly with practices. In addition, a substantial information technology build is required to allow for data sharing between Anthem and the practices. The company, he added, provides significant resources to providers to help with the transformation and to develop the necessary infrastructure and knowledge base to provide high-quality care for their seriously ill patients.

Debono also described Anthem's program, which is still under development, for expanded hospice access. This will include changing the prognosis requirement to 12 months and allow for disease-modifying therapy to continue along with hospice care. Debono said that Anthem anticipates there will be quality improvements on measures such as advance care planning, less aggressive care near the end of life, lower emergency department utilization, and fewer hospitalizations.[16]

In considering ways to optimize palliative care for its members, Debono explained that Anthem examined the barriers to palliative care from a number of perspectives. For example, patients might say that nobody has talked to them about palliative care or that there are no palliative care clinics nearby. Debono said patients also worry about the cost of care or blame their physicians for sending them to the emergency department whenever they get sick. Fear of what it might mean to enroll in palliative care can be a barrier to enrollment.

From a provider's perspective, the perceived extra time needed to deal with patients receiving palliative care can be a barrier, and as with patients, so can the lack of nearby palliative care clinics or teams. Physicians may worry that referring a patient to palliative care might cause them to lose hope.

Payers see other issues with palliative care, said Debono. One issue is that so few Americans have completed advance directives, which results in people often getting aggressive care they do not want (Rao et al., 2014). Another issue is that seriously ill people are not getting the full benefit of hospice, with the average length of stay remaining far below the available 6 months (CMS, 2017c). A third issue is the lack of a central team to help patients navigate through their problems in addition to the symptoms of their illness, including medical bills, anticipatory grief, and caregiving.

To address these issues, Anthem looked at several outpatient palliative care models, each with its own limitations. Primary palliative care, which

---

[16] For further information, see http://www.ehcca.com/presentations/palliativesummit1/wade_ms3.pdf (accessed January 3, 2018).

uses primary care providers or specialists such as oncologists or cardiologists, requires that practitioners and staff receive extensive training. It is also time intensive and not conducive to busy outpatient clinics, said Debono. Primary palliative care also requires resources to develop and staff a primary care team that many practices may not have. Nonetheless, primary palliative care would be a good fit with alternative payment models for care coordination if a practice achieves quality metrics.

Another model uses community-based specialty palliative care. Debono explained that few communities have palliative care specialists, and for communities that do, their palliative care specialists are dedicated to inpatient consulting or hospice work. Fully funding a comprehensive palliative care team is difficult for hospices and hospitals, said Debono, though there is potential for ACOs or large health care systems to enter into a value-based payment model using their own practitioners. This approach, he added, is not easily generalizable to all types of practices.

Third-party organizations that implement palliative care solutions represent a third model. These organizations are staffed with specialty trained professionals—they leverage board-certified palliative medicine physicians and provide different options for 24/7 access to care, including telehealth, home based, and clinic based. Debono said these organizations have been willing to participate in value-based payment models with quality measures and cost-of-care metrics, and they have demonstrated that they can scale palliative care, which he said is an important development.

In closing, Debono predicted his organization will likely adopt an approach that is a hybrid of the models he described. He noted, for example, that large health systems, academic medical centers, and ACOs may want to enter into value-based payment models in which they are responsible for quality and cost and use their own practitioners. Independent practices, for their part, may want to develop their own primary palliative care approach and cultivate novel value-based payment models based initially on achieving quality metrics. Third-party organizations may provide a scalable outpatient solution across markets, across geographic regions, and across different-sized medical practices with reimbursement tied to value-based payment models.

### Lessons from CMS Demonstration Projects

The beneficiary population that CMS serves through its Medicare and Medicaid programs is becoming increasingly complex, noted Shari Ling, deputy chief medical officer in the Center for Clinical Standards and

Quality at CMS, and the agency is fully aware of the implications of this for the care and services that its beneficiaries require. As a payer, this is reflected in the new billing codes CMS has developed for advance care planning, chronic care, cognitive impairment, and care transition. The agency is still learning how these codes are being used, and that information will provide some guidance as to the specific care services being delivered. The challenge, she said, is ensuring that the services delivered are those that the beneficiaries need.

To provide broader context, Ling listed CMS's new goals, which include empowering patients and doctors to make decisions about health care; supporting innovative approaches to improving quality, accessibility, and affordability; and improving the customer experience. She noted the importance of the workshop discussions in terms of informing decision making. The current administration, she added, is ushering in a new era of state flexibility, local leadership, and partnership, with the federal government creating opportunities and, to some extent, developing infrastructure. Commenting on the community work discussed at the workshop, she added that there is an opportunity now for state and local entities to take the lead in developing innovative programs that improve quality, accessibility, and affordability, and go beyond what CMS would normally pay for, which are individual fee-for-service encounters for individual conditions. Ling acknowledged that the challenge CMS faces is trying to fit serious and often complex illnesses into a benefit category defined by prognosis.

CMS's statutory requirements under the Medicare Access and Children's Health Insurance Plan Reauthorization Act of 2015 (MACRA)[17] provide the opportunity to develop and test alternative payment models. The challenge here, said Ling, is to think about how those models will improve outcomes for beneficiaries with serious illness. Contained within MACRA is a merit-based incentive program that requires CMS to include cost in the construct, said Ling. She noted there are emerging opportunities to define and provide the best information possible to ensure that care decisions are aligned with goals of care.

In reviewing the evolving portfolio of demonstration projects, Ling looks at the specific purpose of each project in the context of under what authority they are taking place, the constraints and limitations associated

---

[17] MACRA was signed into law on April 16, 2015. See https://www.cms.gov/Medicare/Quality-Initiatives-Patient-Assessment-Instruments/Value-Based-Programs/MACRA-MIPS-and-APMs/MACRA-MIPS-and-APMs.html (accessed January 22, 2018).

with that authority, and whether any opportunities exist to interpret the requirement under that authority. Each demonstration project, she said, defines the specific practice characteristics, expectations, and metrics for quality and the care experience, and each model addresses payment differently and will provide important lessons for CMS as these projects move forward.

The Independence at Home[18] demonstration project, for example, is testing the hypothesis that providing appropriate care at home will result in greater continuity of care and reveal important insights into the barriers individuals face related to their home environment. This demonstration will have to meet practice-specific minimum savings requirements relative to targeted expenditures, with adjustments for the clinical complexity of a provider's patients, including a provision for frailty, said Ling. While CMS also has authority through the Improving Medicare Post-Acute Care Transformation Act of 2014 (IMPACT)[19] to measure mobility functions, self-care functions, and cognition, it has not had the opportunity yet to translate that authority into hospitals or the outpatient setting. The first 2 years of the program, said Ling, have produced more than $32 million in savings, or approximately $3,000 per beneficiary per year, and resulted in $16 million in shared savings going to practices that met savings and quality goals (CMS, 2017a).

Ling explained another demonstration project, the Medicare Care Choices model,[20] which tests the hypothesis that allowing acute care services to be concurrent with hospice will increase hospice use. Ling noted that early data show that 77 percent of patients in this program elect the hospice benefit when discharged from the hospital.

Ling explained that one lesson CMS has learned from its capitation payment model demonstration, Comprehensive Primary Care Plus (CPC Plus),[21] is that shared savings is not a sufficient incentive by itself to improve patient-centered care and that quality of care metrics also must be included

---

[18] For more information, see https://innovation.cms.gov/initiatives/independence-at-home (accessed January 22, 2018).

[19] For more information, see https://www.cms.gov/Medicare/Quality-Initiatives-Patient-Assessment-Instruments/NursingHomeQualityInits/Downloads/Proposed-Measure-Specifications-for-FY17-SNF-QRP-NPRM.pdf (accessed January 22, 2018).

[20] For more information, see https://innovation.cms.gov/initiatives/Medicare-Care-Choices (accessed January 22, 2018).

[21] The CPC Plus demonstration was authorized by Section 3021 of the Patient Protection and Affordable Care Act and is being conducted by the Centers for Medicare & Medicaid

in the incentives. Another lesson is that CMS needs to be able to pay up front for the delivery of comprehensive care services to give practices some latitude to move from a fee-for-service mentality. What would be helpful going forward, said Ling, is to have the ability to define what qualifies as having a serious illness better, perhaps in terms of function and functional limitations, so that practices and systems could better target those individuals who need more than routine care.

### BSWH's Journey Toward Value in Serious Illness Care

Robert Fine, clinical director in the Baylor Scott & White Health's (BSWH's) Office of Clinical Ethics and Palliative Care, described the experience of his organization—the largest not-for-profit health care system in Texas—as it navigates the transition from fee-for-service toward value-based care for people with serious illness. Fine explained that lessons learned from earlier experience—notably that financial incentives must align—have guided the organization's ongoing palliative care journey. This journey began in 2004, with what Fine refers to as "palliative care 1.0" providing acute death and dying services in 5 of the 10 acute care hospitals in its system at the time. This effort produced limited cost savings data and system administrators were reluctant to expand this service because of its cost.

Fine continued to describe his organization's journey with "palliative care 2.0," which began in 2010. At that time, BSWH administrators, realizing that value-based reimbursement was coming, knew they had to address non-beneficial and unwanted treatment, and decided to reinvest in palliative medicine. BSWH began hiring full-time palliative medicine physicians and advanced practice registered nurses and opened programs in 14 hospitals and 5 outpatient clinics. This new effort focused on seriously ill patients in the hospital, and targeted patients with cancer and congestive heart failure. This effort produced better cost savings data than BSWH's first attempt at palliative care.

Fine pointed out that BSWH's current iteration, "palliative care 3.0," includes more robust specialty palliative care teams and an ongoing initiative in primary palliative care. This effort also focuses on improving communication skills using techniques developed by Ariadne Labs' Communication in Serious Illness project. BSWH has embedded those tools into its

---

Services. See https://innovation.cms.gov/initiatives/comprehensive-primary-care-plus (accessed January 22, 2018).

two major electronic medical record systems. It uses a systematic approach to train providers to use the conversation script and other parts of this tool.

BSWH's current initiative in palliative care was spurred by leadership mandating the creation of robust palliative care teams in each of the system's hospitals, Fine explained. Moreover, they decided to link part of the executive incentive plan not only to build palliative care teams, but to support those teams to ensure specific outcome measures are met.

At the time of the 2.0 effort, BSWH already had high enrollment in hospice, and leadership was doubtful that expanding palliative care would produce additional savings. However, in working with an economist, the BSWH team realized that palliative care did produce savings, but only for those who died while still in the hospital or who entered the program within 9 days of discharge. They also learned that late consults, or consults after more than 9 days of hospitalization, were bad for patients and families because they were not getting the services they needed, and bad for the financial model within which BSWH was trying to develop palliative care.

Other lessons, Fine explained, were that primary diagnosis matters when promoting the program to patients and the greatest cost savings occurred in hospitals with more complete palliative care teams. Fine noted that the program does not turn down patients with diagnoses other than cancer or congestive heart failure, but it does focus more directly on those patients. Today, for example, any patient coming to Baylor University Medical Center to receive a left ventricular assist device or heart transplant meets with the palliative care team for what BSWH calls "preparedness planning."

Fine further emphasized the importance of staying on top of finances. He explained that by entering each hospital's data into the Center to Advance Palliative Care's Impact Calculator,[22] the direct cost savings can be identified and used to remind hospital administrators that cost savings are the same as generating income from procedures.

BSWH's palliative care journey has taught them that hospice is the gold standard for end-of-life care, and is essential, but not sufficient by itself to achieve all of the needed improvements in serious illness care. Similarly, they have realized that having a robust clinical ethics program establishes a moral foundation on which the system expects staff to operate when caring for seriously ill patients. Such a program is essential, but is not sufficient to meet the practical needs of patients, family, or staff.

Palliative care, when appropriately managed, provides significant direct

---

[22] See https://www.capc.org/impact-calculator (accessed January 3, 2018).

cost savings and multiple evidence-based benefits to patients and families, noted Fine. Realizing those benefits requires the health system to make some commitments, including external validation of quality. Fine pointed out that BSWH relies on the Joint Commission certification process for that validation. Additionally, an organization needs to commit to robust data collection. Fine said BSWH collects data on 48 items at every hospital with 100 or more adult beds in its system. These include measures of timeliness of service, care planning, advance directives, and palliation and symptoms outcomes, particularly for pain improvement. Third, there must be a commitment to provide quality support to families, and particularly to children of seriously ill adults, something most programs do not do, said Fine. BSWH now has child life specialists who can serve the children of seriously ill adults.

In closing, Fine emphasized that health systems cannot fund comprehensive primary- and specialty-level palliative care from professional revenue alone. "Cost savings are essential," explained Fine. He believes that value-based payment will be better able to support palliative care, and noted that the transition to value-based payment is complicated and they "are not fully there yet." Specialty palliative care is more challenging to finance in smaller institutions, he added. This is partly because, while palliative care is team based, only physicians and advance practice registered nurses can charge for their services. In addition, despite Medicare's new advance care planning codes, current reimbursement policies do not adequately cover the time involved. Fine cited the key role of a BSWH senior leader who supported building the program and providing incentives to other leaders to do so. "He believed that it is absolutely essential to being prepared for value-based reimbursement," Fine explained. In closing, Fine suggested that payers, both public and private, should reward organizations and providers who demonstrate palliative care competency and quality. He emphasized that value-based payment by itself will not address all of the challenges of expanding palliative care.

### Discussion

After the second session's presentations on financing and payment innovations, Paz opened the discussion by asking the panel what they would describe as the key outcome measures needed to define the quality of the serious illness programs and align that care with value-based reimbursement. Fine explained that because Baylor focuses on patient care planning, creating new advance directives, getting the appropriate changes and code statuses, decreasing the number of attempted, non-beneficial CPRs, and tracking symptom outcomes are very important, despite the variability across hospital campuses. Popiel then added that beyond those metrics, the alignment of the experience of the patients, their caregivers, and their families is also important. However, he noted, the quality of that experience is hard to quantify beyond a typical satisfaction score.

Teresa Lee of VNA Health Group pointed out that her organization is still learning lessons from their participation in the Medicare Care Choices Model and CPC Plus. She noted that although CPC Plus was not originally intended for home care medicine, clinicians are able to innovate because they "have the funds up front [and are able] to make investments" in innovative practices and quality measures. In working with the Medicare Care Choices Model, Lee noted that the program's largest challenge was that payment was not sufficient to provide hospice and all curative treatments comprehensively.

Allison Silvers from the Center to Advance Palliative Care explained that her organization is working to ensure sufficient compensation for the time providers need to attend to the seriously ill. Silvers asked the panel whether there is additional work to be done in terms of investing in bringing the health system up to speed, enhancing the skills that providers need, and whether payers would pay for that training. Popiel responded that Cambia's work is only beginning to scratch the surface "in terms of education and support" for network providers, regardless of whether they are in a "value-based payment arrangement or [a] broader PPO [preferred provider organization] network." He believes there is more to be done, and that the next steps should involve more intensive collaboration and training. Debono agreed, explaining that Anthem "envision[s] a situation in which [the clinicians, staff, and practice] are participating in some sort of value-based payment model and the payer participates in training the practice." Chirico posited that "that methodology [may not] be any better with an insurance-backed concept of education because of the expertise." Ling responded, "practices are learning to redesign themselves" and that the Transforming Clinical Practice Initiative,[23] as an example, is helping to understand the costs and to inform the services that need to be delivered.

Becky Shipp of the Sheridan Group wondered from the "view [of] the

---

[23] For more information, see https://innovation.cms.gov/initiatives/Transforming-Clinical-Practices (accessed March 19, 2018).

field, are these programs working?" To give context, she explained that there are many state-based programs, but many are not available in every state. Dr. Ling explained that the programs have provided access to services, but that the challenge is to determine consistent measures, such as quality, in order to evaluate these programs in a rigorous fashion. She then turned to Ellen Blackwell, also of CMS, who explained that "programs that support home and community services and institutional transition work" have made it easier for states in the Medicaid program to support such services. She explained that over the past few decades, there has been a "complete rebalancing of the system" where more than half of Medicaid patients receiving long-term care do so in a community setting.

## VIEW FROM CONGRESS

Senator Ron Wyden (D-OR), the ranking member of the Senate Committee on Finance, opened his remarks by noting that on September 26, 2017, the Senate unanimously passed a bill to transform Medicare with a focus on chronic illness, one of the three areas—long-term care and end-of-life care being the other two—that drive much of Medicare spending. Ten years ago, Wyden explained, passage of the CHRONIC Care Act would have been on the front page of every newspaper in the United States because it is a truly transformative policy. The reason why this bill is so important, Wyden noted, is that both parties—and he emphasized both parties—had not fully grasped what Medicare has become, which is insurance to cover chronic illness. Passage of the CHRONIC Care Act, said Senator Wyden, updates the Medicare guarantee so that people with chronic illness have more access to telemedicine and non-physician providers, or to someone who coordinates their care and helps them to navigate the "byzantine" U.S. health care system. His hope, now, is that the House of Representatives will pass this bill in some form.

The next area of reform, Senator Wyden explained, needs to be around long-term care, much of which Medicaid pays for in the United States. Repealing the ACA would set reform efforts back to zero, he pointed out, adding that he hopes that instead of going backward, policy makers will "figure out some fresh approaches to financing a bigger role for long-term care under Medicare." Only after that will the focus come to end-of-life care, which has already been the subject of intense debate in Congress, during which the term "death panels" became a rallying cry for those who wanted to defeat the ACA. Senator Wyden noted that one provision in the

ACA was the change in hospice policy that allows someone to have curative therapy without giving up the hospice benefit.

He concluded his remarks by stating that the nation is already spending enough money on health care. What needs to happen, he said, is for the nation to spend that money in the right places. Doing so will depend on providing real value to patients and families and on increasing transparency and accountability in an industry that has virtually no transparency or accountability today.

Representative Phil Roe (R-TN), chair of the House Committee on Veterans' Affairs and a self-proclaimed "country doctor" who practiced medicine in Tennessee for 31 years before being elected to Congress, spoke to the workshop audience as a physician rather than as a politician. He recounted how in the past 3 years he had lost his wife and best friend to cancer, and his mother to cardiac arrest. He also recalled, as a physician, telling a patient that there was nothing more to do for them other than make the end of their life comfortable was the hardest thing he has ever done in his life. For him, improving end-of-life care is not about saving money, but about caring for patients, and improving care for patients with serious illness, and is about spending more time with the patient and less time entering data into an electronic health record (EHR).

In Representative Roe's view, health care should not be political. The focus, he said, should be on providing quality care for patients and deciding whether policies are enabling or hindering that. He agreed with Senator Wyden that there is enough money in the health care system today to deliver quality care to every American, if done properly. One conversation that America must have, though, is on planning for the end of life. "Nobody wants to think about dying or having a chronic illness that incapacitates them in some way, but it is a conversation that we as a country need to have," said Representative Roe. "This is not about left or right. This is about people. This is about doing the right thing for patients." He then mentioned that he is one of the co-sponsors of the Patient Choice and Quality Care Act,[24] a bill that aims to improve the delivery of palliative care and better

---

[24] The Patient Choice and Quality Care Act of 2017, introduced on June 6, 2017, would allow for a CMMI demonstration of Advanced Illness Coordination, giving patients with multiple and chronic conditions access to palliative care, psychosocial support, and other home-based services, as well as fund further education around advance care planning. For more information, see https://www.congress.gov/bill/115th-congress/house-bill/2797 (accessed March 14, 2018).

reflect patient choice. In closing, he encouraged workshop participants to talk to their representatives and senators about supporting this bill.

## EXPLORING FINANCING AND PAYMENT INNOVATIONS: CHALLENGES, IMPACTS, AND LESSONS FROM GLOBAL BUDGETING ARRANGEMENTS

In her introduction to the workshop's third session, Cheryl Phillips, president and chief executive officer of SNP Alliance, pointed out that new financing and payment strategies are needed because the volume-based, fee-for-service model has not worked well for individuals with complex care needs, including those with serious illness. She described SNPs as a type of Medicare and Medicaid managed care targeting high-risk, high-cost, vulnerable populations. These populations include those who are eligible for both Medicare and Medicaid, individuals receiving long-term institutional care as deemed by the state, and those who have serious chronic health issues. Phillips noted that these plans "align policy, payment, and practice to serve these high-risk, high-need populations." She juxtaposed these plans against the managed care plans in the 1980s and 1990s, which Phillips said, "were rarely managed and had less to do with care." By contrast, she said, today's managed care or global payment models seem to be able to truly target and provide better care for high-risk, high-need, and high-cost individuals.

### Financing Quality Care for Serious Illness at Kaiser Permanente

The "secret sauce" that enables Kaiser Permanente to deliver high-quality care, explained Annet Arakelian, executive director of Medicare strategy and care delivery at Kaiser, is the way it has aligned its revenues and expenses. Kaiser's revenue comes from the Kaiser Foundation health plan that collects premiums from groups, individual members, and some prospective contracts with government payers. Expenses go through a hospital service agreement with Kaiser Foundation hospitals and a capitated medical service agreement with the Permanente Medical Groups that employ the physicians who work at Kaiser hospitals and clinics. The hospitals and foundation are nonprofit organizations, while the medical groups are for-profit agencies with their own board of directors and governance processes. Incentives are aligned across the hospitals, health plan, and medical groups on quality metrics, as well as financial and regulatory initiatives.

Susan Wang, regional lead for shared decision making at the Southern California Permanente Medical Group, explained that Kaiser's approach to comprehensive financing of serious illness care begins with a population health perspective, which stems from the capitated arrangement that features a fixed payment per person enrolled in its medical groups. "Because we are capitated, we are accountable for our entire membership, it behooves us to touch our patients at every opportunity," said Wang. When patients contact Kaiser for any reason, preventive health and disease management reminders are either reviewed by protocol or automatically displayed in the EHR, helping individuals get care for which they are due. In addition, the EHR includes a systematic screen to catch "misses," which means that if the clinic staff missed a particular care item at the time of a member's visit, the system provides alerts to reach back to the member. This integrated system, which Kaiser calls Complete Care, provides evidence-based screening, disease detection, and optimal disease management. Since its inception in 2004, Complete Care has enabled Kaiser to improve its Healthcare Effectiveness Data and Information Set (HEDIS) scores by an average of 13 percent across 51 HEDIS measures and save millions of dollars in the process, said Wang.

One successful component of Complete Care is its online personal action plan, an email-based outreach tool that links to a personalized plan for members and targets a member's pre-office encounter to prepare them for their upcoming visit. Members who use this tool show a high rate of care gap closure, said Wang (Kaiser Permanente, 2013). The tool also allows patients to book appointments for services like mammograms and A1C testing without requiring a physician-based office encounter to do so and improves the efficiency of care management (Henry et al., 2016). For example, Kaiser launched an initiative in December 2016 to reduce colon cancer mortality by 50 percent over 10 years through more intensive screening and by reducing variations in treatment for advanced colorectal cancer. As a result, online tool users ordered 13,000 fecal immunochemical test kits, a screening test for colorectal cancer, and returned 68 percent of them. Over the first 4 years of this initiative, colorectal cancer mortality declined by 2.5 per 100,000 Kaiser members (Henry et al., 2016).

SureNet, another Complete Care component, is designed to augment medication safety and disease detection by using protocols built into Kaiser's EHR. For example, the program reviews laboratory results to look for issues that might be overlooked by a primary care physician, such as gross hematuria in a urine sample. In one sampling, the program called for nearly 600 follow-up cystoscopies after screening 2,200 urine samples, which led to the detection of 17 cancers and 41 other clinically significant abnormalities. Another SureNet evaluation focuses on certain drug–drug interactions that can cause adverse outcomes. In one 2-year pilot program, SureNet alerts potentially avoided 22 emergency department visits and 44 hospitalizations, saving Kaiser $2.14 for every $1 spent running this program (Spence et al., 2011).

In terms of inpatient medicine, Kaiser has been able to reduce hospital use by approximately 30 percent over the past decade, which Wang said has translated into patients receiving higher quality care in the home setting, as well as billions of dollars in cost savings for the entire enterprise. Patients who are hospitalized benefit from Kaiser's integrated inpatient quality management system, a patient flow oversight model that aligns department processes to improve the timeliness and appropriateness of patient care through enhanced provider communication and the identification and removal of system barriers to care. According to Wang, this program has been shown to improve the quality of patient care at the bedside, optimize the patient care experience, and produce marked cost savings.[25]

In thinking about the total health of its members, at least 80 percent of what affects patient health is associated with the social determinants of health. According to Wang, a pilot project contacted 3,000 Kaiser members who were predicted to be in the top 1 percent of high users and assessed and addressed various social needs. Arakelian said a preliminary analysis found a potential impact on cost and usage from addressing social needs.[26]

The final program Wang discussed was Kaiser's Life Care Planning System, which she called a systematic approach to advance care planning based on respecting choices. This program segments members into three groups—healthy adults and those with stable chronic illness, adults of any age with progressive advanced illness, and adults of any age whose death within the next 12 to 18 months would not be surprising—and targets them with actions appropriate for each group's current situation. The healthy group, for example, is directed toward online life care planning and class-based discussions for members and family members. Activities focus on naming a health care agent and thinking about contingencies for future events. For the progressive advanced illness group, which accounts for 16 percent of Kaiser's members, the focus is on disease-specific shared decision

---

[25] Information was unpublished/in press at the time of this proceedings' publication.

[26] Information was unpublished/in press at the time of this proceedings' publication.

making, while the final group, accounting for 8 percent of Kaiser's members, discusses specific goals and wishes for life-prolonging treatment and intensity of treatment and creates associated medical orders. According to Wang, some half million members have engaged in this program.[27] Kaiser has intentionally not used cost or usage as a measure, focusing instead on quality, Wang said.

In closing, Wang said that Kaiser's philosophy regarding its members with serious illness is that they are more likely to experience transitions in care, and coordinated, patient-centered care is critical to producing the best outcomes. With its own palliative care and hospice capabilities, it is not uncommon for a single physician to be able to follow a member from site to site as they experience those transitions, which she said is what helps the organization optimize care for its members.

## Global Payment Arrangements for Serious Illness Care in Massachusetts

Massachusetts has seen high rates of adoption of global payment arrangements across payers and programs, said Anna Gosline, senior director of health policy and strategic initiatives at Blue Cross Blue Shield of Massachusetts (BCBSMA) (see Figure 3). The strongest adoption has been among commercial plans, with approximately 40 percent of commercial members receiving care under a global payment plan (see Figure 4). Nearly 25 percent of the members in Medicaid managed plans and Medicaid fee-for-service plans receive care under global payment arrangements (Center for Health Information and Analysis, 2017).

Gosline explained that the transition to global payment arrangements in Massachusetts began in 2006, when the state passed its universal coverage law. Within 18 months of passage, virtually everyone in the state was insured, creating significant cost pressure in a state that already had the highest per capita spending on health care in the nation.

At the time, leaders at BCBSMA realized that the biggest contribution it could make in terms of improving cost and quality was to change the way the organization paid for care, and worked to develop a global payment model. Gosline explained that Massachusetts General Hospital began participating in the Medicare Care Management demonstration project for high-cost beneficiaries in 2009. Around that same time, the first Alternative

---

[27] Information was unpublished/in press at the time of this proceedings' publication.

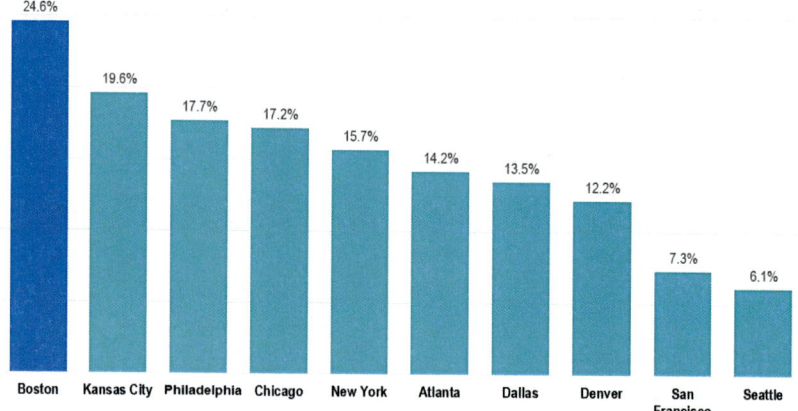

**FIGURE 3** Share of regional Medicare beneficiaries cared for under the Medicare Share Savings ACO program.
NOTE: ACO = accountable care organization.
SOURCES: As presented by Anna Gosline and Vicki Jackson, November 29, 2017; Center for Health Information and Analysis, 2017.

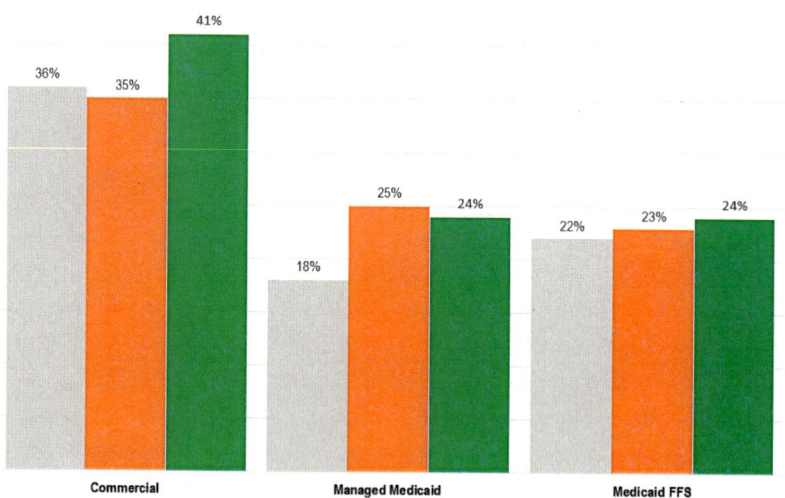

**FIGURE 4** Share of members whose care was paid for under a global payment arrangement.
NOTE: FFS = fee for service.
SOURCES: As presented by Anna Gosline and Vicki Jackson, November 29, 2017; CMS, 2018.

Quality Contracts (AQCs) were rolled out in the health maintenance organization market, which accounts for about half of the commercial market in the state. Partners Healthcare—the umbrella system to which Massachusetts General Hospital belongs—joined the AQC program and became a Medicare Pioneer ACO 1 year later. By 2013, 85 percent of Massachusetts physicians were participating in the AQC program. In 2016, BCBSMA expanded global payments to its preferred provider organization (PPO) plan, with Partners Healthcare joining the BCBSMA PPO model later that same year and becoming a Medicare "Next Gen" ACO (BCBSMA, 2015).

BCBSMA's AQC program includes a global budget that covers all medical services using a shared risk model that adjusts for health status based on historical claims. The program includes quality incentives for ambulatory and hospital settings based on nationally accepted measures that provide the potential for a significant earnings boost. Its 5-year contract helps sustain partnerships and supports ongoing investments. Gosline noted that as the financial model evolved, the systems that performed better on their quality measures were eligible to receive additional shared savings and pay back less if they had a shared loss.

Quality results under the AQC model have surpassed the HEDIS national average for adult chronic care and pediatric care (Song et al., 2014). Gosline pointed out that during a time when HEDIS measures on adult health outcomes were stagnant, AQC groups realized significant improvements. An evaluation by investigators at Harvard Medical School during the first 4 years of the program found accelerating medical claims cost savings (Song et al., 2014). Gosline pointed out that the program had grown to include such a large percentage of the health systems in Massachusetts that this study had to use out-of-state controls (CMS, 2018).

Given that these results focused on a commercially insured population, where the number of people with serious and advancing illnesses is relatively small on a percentage basis, the question arose as to whether the AQC model offered sufficient incentives to produce the same results to provide better care for individuals with serious illness at lower cost. To answer that question, BCBSMA worked with Ariadne Labs to implement a primary palliative care program in two different systems in the state. This effort, said Gosline, works hand in hand with her organization's policy and community efforts, which established a statewide coalition of approximately 85 organizations working together to improve care for those with serious illness. "By no means do we have all the answers, but we understand the power of payers talking together to send similar messages into the marketplace," said Gosline.

Vicki Jackson, chief of the division of palliative care and geriatric medicine at Massachusetts General Hospital, discussed her organization's home-based palliative care pilot program. The program grew out of the realization that many individuals who could benefit from palliative care, such as Patricia Bencivenga, are too ill to engage in a longitudinal medical relationship with their provider and are not eligible for hospice. The pilot is embedded in the organization's ACO and, like all seriously ill patients in the Partners system, individuals in the pilot are assigned a nurse care manager who identifies patients with unmet palliative needs that would be better served by a home-based program. The nurse care managers, Jackson explained, have a wealth of resources available to them, including psychiatrists, pharmacy advisors, and community resource specialists who have money available to cover non-medical expenses, such as installing an air conditioner in the home of someone with COPD.

The population of patients referred to the pilot fall into three categories, said Jackson. In one group are individuals who should have been referred to hospice several months earlier, and most of these individuals do transition to hospice after one or two home visits. Those in the second group are highly symptomatic and typically have multiple chronic conditions. After engaging with the program and having their needs met, individuals in this group eventually transition into the first group or the third group. The third group includes patients who are more stable and may not yet require hospice. Rather, this group would realistically need a less intensive model of home-based care to meet their needs. Now, 4 years into the program, Jackson and her colleagues realized they have a cohort of 15 to 20 individuals, mostly women over age 90, with multiple chronic conditions and significant cognitive impairment who were stable and not eligible for hospice. The decision was made to keep this small cohort enrolled in the program and continue with the care plan, though with fewer home visits.

Jackson noted that two evaluations of the program have shown a savings of $1,351 per member, per month during the last 6 months of life. Most of the savings result from fewer hospitalizations and decreased expenses during hospital stays, and from increasing hospice use and length of stay on hospice. The net benefit per patient to the ACO, after deducting shared savings with CMS and the cost of the program, is $2,696.[28] Jackson

---

[28] Information was unpublished/in press at the time of this proceedings' publication.

said that is not a huge savings, making it important to think about how best to manage different populations of people with serious illness. Jackson explained that what is needed to care for a person who is incredibly short of breath is different from what a person who is stable needs until they have aspiration issues related to pneumonia, for example. "We have to be nimble and think about that," said Jackson. Massachusetts General Hospital has expanded the program to cover most of the greater Boston area and is finding that the geographic issues are significant. "Making sure we have the right people in the right places is a tricky piece," she added.

In closing, Jackson said an important lesson to take away from this initiative is the need to have a convincing argument that addresses key issues for leadership. Given that the margins are not large, it was important for her to ask for something reasonable that was the right size for that return. Another lesson was that it will be necessary to be flexible and ready to adapt any program as it progresses. She also emphasized the importance of relationships. For example, as the leader of an academic medical center, her relationship with Gosline, a leader at a payer, has been incredibly helpful for developing and improving her program. Gosline agreed and said the input she has received from Jackson has helped her think about more targeted incentives to help other systems address their own internal cost structure. For example, the AQC now includes directed payment for community-based palliative care, something she did not envision happening and probably would not have happened had she not been able to interact with Jackson to understand the nature of the financing that allowed her program to be successful.

### Complex Care Management at OptumHealth

One area of OptumHealth's strategy to establish sustainable financing for serious illness care is to focus on transitions as a means of reducing readmissions, explained Gregory James, senior medical director at OptumCare, a division of OptumHealth. Readmissions cost Medicare more than $17 billion annually in avoidable costs, said James. For context, he noted that one in five elderly patients is readmitted to the hospital within 30 days of discharge, that 40 percent of Medicare beneficiaries are discharged from the hospital to a post-acute setting, and that half of those individuals enter an SNF (Mor et al., 2010).

The program Transitions to Skilled Nursing Facility, developed by OptumCare, manages the transition to SNFs and assigns a nurse practitioner or physician assistant to each patient when they enter the nursing facility. There is an initial visit or contact with the patient within 24 hours of entering the nursing facility. This initial meeting is designed to focus on discharge planning, care coordination, and providing quality care. The assigned clinician makes frequent visits to monitor the patient for changes in condition, then develops a care coordination plan in collaboration with facility staff, family support caregivers, and the patient's primary care physician. When discharged, the patient is referred to a post-discharge program to ensure there is a successful transition to home that reduces the need for readmissions.

Within 1 year of instituting this post-acute management program, James described how a partnership between OptumCare and an organization in the Midwest had produced significant improvements, including a 20 percent reduction in length of stay in the nursing home and a 52 percent reduction in readmissions to the hospital. The same program instituted in partnership with another organization, said James, produced a 43 percent reduction in length of stay and a 33 percent reduction in readmissions. Both programs served a Medicare Advantage population. The potential cost savings to a health plan from implementing the Transitions to Skilled Nursing Facility program and cutting readmissions by 20 percent would be approximately $80,000, while the savings from reducing length of stay by 20 percent would be approximately $205,000, James said.[29]

James explained that optimizing the length of stay for patients—looking at the patients and ensuring that they are going home at the appropriate time—has been an effective cost-saving approach. "One of the primary ways we do that is by starting discharge planning on day one," he said. Starting discharge planning early enables tasks to be completed such as scheduling doctor appointments and reviewing, planning, and even delivering medication to the home. Furthermore, it enables home assessments to be completed before the patient is discharged or, as is the case for 5 to 10 percent of patients, transferred to long-term care. In addition to saving money, this program improves quality measures by closing gaps in care and improving patient and family satisfaction. This is largely due to the increased attention that patients get from their nurse practitioner or physician assistant, and the time they spend on advance care planning.

---

[29] Information is courtesy of Optum's Analytics Division and was unpublished/in press at the time of this proceedings' publication.

Another OptumCare program is the Institutional Special Needs Plan (I-SNP), which delivers coordinated care for Medicare long-term nursing care residents. The program is open to long-term Medicare A and B patients who are not on dialysis, and patients are not restricted to a specific period during which they can enroll in or disenroll from the program, which James said is not typical of this type of program. He noted there are 1.5 million Medicare beneficiaries living in SNFs, and those who do are twice as expensive to care for as the average beneficiary. According to James, more than half of SNF-based Medicare beneficiaries had one or more emergency department visits, compared with 28 percent for non-SNF-based beneficiaries, and 33 percent had at least one hospitalization, compared with 19 percent for non-SNF-based beneficiaries. Currently, only about 3 percent of these SNF residents are enrolled in an institutional special needs Medicare Advantage program.[30]

A broken clinical model, explained James, is what drives the high costs associated with these individuals. Increasingly, he said, more SNFs have dedicated geriatricians who only work in nursing homes. However, much of the care that individuals in these facilities receive is from their primary care physician, with the result that there is often poor coordination of care. Supplying a nurse practitioner to an SNF improves communication and coordination, increases advance care planning, and improves polypharmacy issues that are often not addressed adequately. The nurse practitioner also works on engaging with and educating family members and coordinating any social services the patient needs.

In closing, James pointed out that OptumCare has been delivering this model for 25 years and serves 80 percent of the patients enrolled in this type of program. James said the program reduces costs by 50 percent for its members, and cuts hospitalizations by 40 percent and emergency department visits by nearly 50 percent. Member satisfaction with the plan has been consistently around 98 percent, he added, with a voluntary disenrollment rate of less than 1 percent. Most of those individuals leave the program because they return to the community.[31]

---

[30] Information is courtesy of Optum's Analytics Division and was unpublished/in press at the time of this proceedings' publication.

[31] Information is courtesy of Optum's Analytics Division and was unpublished/in press at the time of this proceedings' publication.

## Discussion

In the discussion session following the presentations, Gosline pointed to a key challenge in developing financing arrangements with commercial plans: the number of members under age 65 with serious illness is relatively small, although the fixed costs of staffing these programs and building capacity can be high. "There needs to be enough volume to create enough shared savings to support those fixed costs on an ongoing basis," she said. The same is true, she said, if she targets financing to support community-based palliative care because as a commercial payer, she will still only cover a small percentage of the patient population. Another challenge, she explained, arises from the lack of good quality measures that can be used to drive attention to these programs. She noted, though, that adding new measures is not likely to win favor from providers, many of whom already feel overwhelmed by existing measures.

Jackson added that staffing these programs with skilled clinicians is a challenge, given that being a good home care clinician is different from being a good geriatrician or palliative care clinician. Phillips agreed that workforce challenges are significant, extending beyond nurses and physicians to include social workers, therapists, case managers, and pharmacists who understand the complexity of serious illness and the need to carefully coordinate care. Gosline said one unanticipated challenge in Massachusetts is that there has been such a high rate of adoption across the state that it is nearly impossible to hire a social work or case manager.

James identified another challenge, which arises from the tension between cutting the length of stay in nursing homes and the fact that nursing homes, for the most part, are paid on a daily rate. This reality makes it important for OptumCare to create shared-savings contracts that incentivize the nursing facility to have the patient leave sooner if appropriate. Wang said that for Kaiser, alternative payment models can be either too restrictive or come too late. For example, California just approved a temporary rule to allow home-based palliative care to be administered under hospice, but Kaiser has been doing this since 2006 of its own accord.

Phillips said that while HEDIS measures are viewed as important for commercial plans and younger populations, they have virtually no meaning for those with serious illness, which goes back to the issue that Gosline raised earlier about the need for quality measures for these types of programs. Gosline pointed out that having measures of patient and family experience would be a good start. For BCBSMA, patient-reported outcome measures are becoming a large part of its global payment arrangement and are now required for cancer and cardiac care beneficiaries. Her organization is working with Ariadne Labs to look at possible patient-reported outcome measures for other serious illness situations that could fit into the workflow and capture patient experience during the clinical encounter. BCBSMA is also looking at developing some type of bereaved family survey, although there are many operational challenges that the organization is working through in partnership with Ariadne Labs, said Gosline. Wang noted that Kaiser is currently rolling out a nationwide bereaved family survey.

James noted that satisfying some of the National Committee for Quality Assurance (NCQA) measures, such as those for breast cancer and colon cancer screening, could put older, seriously ill patients at risk. To NCQA's credit, when officials from OptumCare explained that risks of doing a colonoscopy on a 75-year-old nursing home resident outweigh the benefits, NCQA removed the 66- to 75-year-old group in long-term care nursing facilities from that quality measure.

Jackson pointed out that as her organization has been rolling out its serious illness conversation program, it has relieved its physicians, and particularly its primary care providers, of needing to check the box on certain measures. "It relieved the clinicians just knowing they were not going to be held accountable for things they did not think were important anyway," said Jackson. Wang noted that Kaiser is trying to build palliative care skills with the medical specialties and at the same time is trying to systematize process measures relevant to those specialties.

Phillips asked the panelists if any of their plans have a formal screen for social determinants of health, and if so, whether they use that information to make risk adjustments either for payment or for quality measure performance. Jackson said her program does have a formal screen for social determinants and does use that information for risk adjustment purposes. She noted that a program serving vulnerable elders in the community is going to find that social determinants have a large effect on the health of those individuals. Ignoring them, she added, is one of the core problems in treating individuals with serious illness because it is hard to manage them if they do not have transportation, good housing, caregiving, or adequate nutrition.

Arakelian said that Kaiser has developed a set of 10 questions called "Your Current Life Situation" that will be available to everyone in a Kaiser plan through the EHR to document social needs.[32] What excites her about this survey is that the data it provides may enable some hotspotting regarding certain types of patients that Kaiser can better target for interventions. This statement prompted Phillips to ask James how his program targets beneficiaries to participate in its programs. James responded that for the I-SNP program, the program can only sign up patients in contracted facilities. For its Transitions to SNF program, the nurse practitioner assigned to a facility receives an email notice that there is a new UnitedHealthcare Medicare Advantage Plan[33] beneficiary in their facility.

Rob Saunders of Duke University asked about different quality and cost performance outcomes for hospital-led ACOs versus physician-led ACOs and how financing approaches might be implemented in organizations that have different characteristics and competencies. Gosline responded that in her state there is a wide variety of organizations participating in global payment arrangements. "You can't really predict cost savings and quality measures based on organizational styles," she said.

Referring to the challenge of using historical benchmarks for shared savings programs, workshop participant Phillip Rodgers from the University of Michigan Medical School suggested that perhaps the key is to "look to a place in the future where we value the service and we support it appropriately as opposed to expecting it to save money." He pointed out that "high-performing, efficient systems do not want to participate in those shared savings models because they can't make [them] work for them."

## EXPLORING POTENTIAL REGULATORY AND POLICY CHANGES TO ENSURE HIGH-QUALITY CARE FOR PEOPLE OF ALL AGES WITH SERIOUS ILLNESS

When his father died of cancer in Indiana about a decade ago, Patrick Conway, president and chief executive officer of BCBSNC,[34] was helping to manage his care from hundreds of miles away, even with incredibly well-meaning providers and care teams in place. At one point, he explained, he

---

[32] The questionnaire was launched in January 2016. See https://sirenetwork.ucsf.edu/tools-resources/mmi/kaiser-permanentes-your-current-life-situation-survey (accessed January 23, 2018).

[33] OptumCare and OptumHealth are divisions of UnitedHealthcare.

[34] Conway previously served as CMS's chief medical officer, deputy administrator for Innovation and Quality, and director of CMMI.

had to fly to Indiana to talk to his father's hospitalist, who thought his dad's blood pressure and potassium levels were at dangerous levels and wanted to keep him in the hospital, even though his father preferred to die at home. Conway said this was not a fault of the care teams, but rather a symptom of the systems in place. It also serves to highlight one of the many opportunities to improve care for people with serious illness.

To Conway, serious illness care comes back to patient- and family-centered care, and he stresses to his organization that treating every member as if they are family helps to ensure the organization will succeed in its mission to help improve the health of the people of North Carolina. He acknowledged that training and education of staff will be critical to the organization's success because many clinicians and care teams are at different stages of understanding the importance of serious illness care and how best to provide that care. He applauded the decision of CMS to pay for advance care planning and pointed out that while there is room for improving how the agency pays for serious illness care, the idea of delivering hospice and palliative care services concurrent with so-called curative care is a step in the right direction. Conway stressed, however, that in his view, "We do have to do more in serious illness payment models so we cannot just say we will solve it with ACOs or comprehensive primary care . . . there also have to be very specific payment models focused on serious illness care."

BCBSNC has several initiatives testing approaches to reimbursement, training, care team engagement, and investments in advanced illness care and advanced directives. The organization now has a palliative care advisory group and ongoing palliative care pilot projects, as well as pilots focused on how to provide care coordination for patients with serious illness and their families. Conway explained that his organization's challenge moving forward is to assess the array of care models available and expand those models that are working well.

He recounted one lesson from an experience involving a child with a genetic disorder who he found out had not been getting life-saving medication for 1 month. Fortunately, his team fixed the problem in 40 minutes and then conducted an after-action review that was one of the best he had seen in years. This review found that a customer representative spent 80 minutes on the phone trying to resolve the problem and had no way to escalate the issue effectively. As a result, BCBSNC is now empowering its frontline representatives to treat every member as if they are family and escalate a problem appropriately so that the next child or adult with serious illness has a better care experience.

Conway ended his remarks with a story about caring for a 13-year-old girl with multiple, progressive chronic conditions from which she would never recover. At the time, he was working for CMS and saw patients on the weekends, and during one of those weekends, he had a very difficult conversation with the girl's mother. He took care of this mother and child over several subsequent weekends and then, as sometimes happens with hospital medicine, he lost track of them. One day, while walking through the halls of CMS, he ran into the girl's mother who told him that difficult conversation changed the course of her family's life for the better. Subsequently, she had been inspired to transfer from another federal agency to CMS to work with Conway. That story, explained Conway, underscores the importance of ensuring that care teams have a level of training that enables them to have those conversations and provide the kind of care everyone wants for their families.

## Policy Opportunities

Edo Banach, president and chief executive officer of the National Hospice and Palliative Care Organization, began his remarks with the observation that "despite all our innovations and all the great work at CMS,[35] most people are still getting care from either a 1965 or a 1983 version of Medicare, where the question is whether the care you are getting is medically necessary, or if you are talking about home health, the question is whether there is a skilled need or whether you are homebound, or if you are talking about hospice, the question is whether you have less than 6 months to live." That is the reality, he said, regardless of the discussion about value and person-centered care, and the fact is that most providers still fight those battles every day as they try to deliver the right care for their patients.

As an example of the misalignment within the current system at a time when the focus is supposedly on value, Banach pointed out that it should not be easier for a 94-year-old to get hip replacement surgery paid for by Medicare than to get home attendant services or palliative care. Medicare still considers some of the things that are most valuable to living a fulfilled life to be ancillary unless a patient is on hospice, Banach said. He believes

---

[35] Banach previously served as the deputy director of the Medicare–Medicaid Coordination Office at CMS.

hospice is a good model for the kind of care that Medicare can deliver to the rest of its beneficiaries.

One structural shortcoming of the current Medicare approach that concerns Banach is that the lack of a long-term benefit under Medicare drives many people to impoverish themselves so they can receive long-term care coverage through Medicaid. He predicted that if Medicare provided interdisciplinary, person-centered care long before needing hospice, people would avail themselves of that benefit and use less curative—and expensive—care. His hope is that the Medicare Care Choices program will find this to be true. What is not speculative, though, is that preventing people from having to draw down or hide their assets to get into Medicaid saves the total system money. "That is a structural change related to the relationship between Medicare and Medicaid that we need to look closely at," said Banach.

Although hospice has come a long way in 30 years, it still needs to evolve to focus more on quality of care and on what families need to support the patient, said Banach. At the same time, lessons learned from hospice over those three decades can inform approaches to better care throughout the health care system. He noted that at times of natural disaster, hospice is often called on to provide bereavement counseling to the local population, not as a paid activity, but as a part of the community service that hospice provides. In some parts of the country today, he added, hospice is also providing bereavement counseling to the survivors of the opioid crisis that is ravaging communities. Currently, hospice is in the mode of waiting for the physical manifestation of an ailment to reach a point that an individual is in the final months of life and then provides great interdisciplinary care. Banach wondered if hospice could be more proactive in analyzing how it could support behavioral health and addiction issues before they lead to suicide and death.

Before discussing the work that his organization does to help providers transition to value-based payment, Julian Harris, president of CareAllies, recounted his grandparents' 10-year journey that began with his grandmother's Alzheimer's diagnosis. At that time, his grandfather, who had worked for the U.S. Department of Agriculture and helped raise five children, decided his life mission was to care for his wife. Fortunately, his grandmother was one of the rare individuals who had purchased long-term care insurance when she had been an elementary school teacher, so they were able to have a home health aide come twice per day to help with some of his wife's activities of daily living. In addition, his grandmother was able to engage hospice care. Harris has incredible memories of the time he, his siblings, and the rest of the family spent with the hospice team making sure that his grandmother's last days were the way she would have wanted. Harris shared this story to encourage everyone—when they inevitably find themselves in that same position as a child, grandchild, or spouse—to allow themselves to stay connected with these personal stories because they will shape the way one works and the way one approaches these efforts throughout their lives.

Harris then described how when he was involved in establishing the Medicare–Medicaid dual-eligible demonstration program in Massachusetts, he and his team made a point of engaging the robust advocacy community in the state, which enabled them to engage with a diverse set of stakeholders. What he found particularly interesting was that many of these advocates had already thought about how to coordinate medical care and services and, as a result, were able to provide an understanding about the disconnect between medical services and the long-term services and supports that those with serious illness need to life full lives. As a result, according to Harris, the demonstration project created a staff position specifically to help ensure that the spectrum of long-term services and supports were not disconnected from medical services and to make sure people—including those in the health care system—knew these services and supports were available.

Another lesson learned when setting up the demonstration was that in some cases, people had multiple care coordinators appointed by state agencies, health plans, and even their providers. "There was this cacophony of care coordinators, all trying to do the right thing and all trying to help the patient, but not necessarily coordinating among themselves or even knowing that each other existed," said Harris. Instead of helping, these well-meaning care coordinators often "complicat[ed] the lives of people who already navigated a great deal of complexity." Although the demonstration was not always able to reduce the number of care coordinators, the program made sure they knew of one another and encouraged them to coordinate their efforts.

In terms of financing, an important lesson was that Harris and his colleagues were overly ambitious, in retrospect, about the potential savings. "If you take a population that has been underserved in a fee-for-service model for a significant time and put them in a managed environment, it will take time to achieve savings," said Harris. In some cases, he added, there may be savings, but not as large as expected.

Turning to his current work at CareAllies, Harris said the organization supports practices and health systems covering some 200,000 Medicare Shared Savings program and 500,000 Medicare Advantage beneficiaries, and helps them navigate the transition to value-based payment. One thing he tells his team, many of whom were not trained as physicians, is that they must remember that the providers they are helping were taught how to take care of individual patients. Most physicians, he said, were not taught how to care for a population of 1,500 individuals, some percentage of whom have diabetes or COPD, and they need to learn how to think at both the population and individual levels and how to be responsible for the total cost of care of an individual.

Harris shared that his team has also learned that it needs to teach physicians and nurses how to go into a home and do a risk assessment and to provide primary care in the home. This is a different skill set, said Harris, one that most primary care providers have not been taught. In fact, this is not a skill set appropriate for every primary care physician. Part of CareAllies' role is to develop the right workforce that can best provide care in the home.

Rodney Whitlock, vice president for health policy at ML Strategies, spoke from his experience as a congressional staff member for 21 years. He observed that the path to successfully changing the nature of how health care is provided requires using a continuum of care models—from hangnail to hospice, or cough to coffin, as he put it—that use risk-bearing entities to deliver care. Such an approach will create an ideal alignment to produce optimal outcomes, rather than misalignment in today's system that produces outcomes that "drive us insane every day," said Whitlock.

Getting to a continuum of care model using risk-based entities requires policy change, and that requires convincing a majority of senators and representatives, all of whom are trying to understand health care and a few of whom actually do at the level needed to fully grasp the effects of health care policy. This task is particularly challenging given that there are two groups in Congress with fundamentally different philosophical views of health care. One group believes that by emphasizing universal coverage and ensuring the quality of care is as high as possible, the cost issue will solve itself eventually. The other group looks at the same issue and believes that cost is paramount and must be controlled by any means necessary, which will eventually lead to universal coverage that may include the highest-quality care possible. "When you have two so diametrically opposed views of the approach to health care, finding the common ground for conversation is extraordinarily difficult," said Whitlock. Making it more difficult is the common response that proposed policy changes will "destroy Medicare."

Fortunately, Whitlock added, there are opportunities to look at this issue differently. The Center for Medicare & Medicaid Innovation (CMMI), created as part of the ACA, has the remarkable ability to experiment with different models of care and financing in the Medicare and Medicaid programs without having to get approval or permission from Congress. He noted that from Congress's perspective, this freedom to experiment is extraordinarily offensive, but it is nonetheless effective at testing new ideas and implementing them in Medicare or Medicaid. As an example, Whitlock offered the example of when he worked on a bill for Senator Charles Grassley (R-IA) to create the Diabetes Prevention Program.[36] This program is now being implemented in Medicare, but not because it became law—the Congressional Budget Office said it would cost tens of billions of dollars and not be effective, explained Whitlock. Rather, CMMI believed this program was the right thing to do and had the authority to test the program and then implement it nationally. In closing, Whitlock said the challenge in getting Congress to do something different is to make a case that is so overwhelmingly convincing that Congress will be willing to take a risk, change policy, and try a different approach to delivering high-quality health care to those with serious illness.

**Panel Discussion**

Following their brief remarks, Banach, Conway, Harris, and Whitlock had a lively discussion about policy changes that could incentivize higher quality care for people with serious illness. Banach said he would like to see policies that remove some of the barriers to getting palliative and hospice care, such as eliminating the 6-month limit on hospice and the need to demonstrate on a case-by-case basis that a given service is needed for a Medicare beneficiary. He also wants policy to create a bundle of supports and services that would help prevent a decline in Medicare beneficiaries rather than having to wait for them to decline before providing care, which he said would require providing CMS with more flexibility regarding medical necessity.

Harris said his priorities would include reauthorization of the Children's Health Insurance Program (CHIP) and Dual Eligible Special Needs Plans and for Congress to pass the CHRONIC Care Act that Senator

---

[36] For more information, see https://www.grassley.senate.gov/news/news-releases/grassley-welcomes-success-medicare-diabetes-prevention-pilot-program (accessed March 14, 2018).

Wyden spoke about earlier. He also said he would like to see some creative approaches in terms of accountability for drug spending in Medicare, whether under Part A or Part D. He supports CMS's agenda on administrative simplification, reducing the paperwork burden for providers, and being thoughtful about measures.

Whitlock shared that in his view, "Every day that we move farther and farther away from classic fee for service is a good day." He would like to see the payment structure shift to focus on appropriate usage. In response, Banach offered an example of the difference between use and appropriate use: A hospice may discharge a patient who has lived longer than 6 months to avoid an audit. That patient might then end up in the emergency department and subsequently hospitalized, however, costing Medicare much more money than if that patient had been allowed to stay in hospice. Banach pointed out that the silos involved in providing fee-for-service care—hospice in one silo, home health in another, and so on—often lead to significantly greater Medicare spending. CMS is aware of this problem, but is constrained by the way Congress wrote the Medicare law, added Banach.

Harris said that he was not sure that a statute was needed to address that problem and pointed out that innovative companies are advocating for the ability to have home-based primary care and home-based pre-palliative care reimbursed in Medicare fee for service, which he supports. In fact, Harris said, many venture-backed companies are trying to disrupt the Medicare fee-for-service space, and he would like to see policy that would enable these private companies to have their models scaled if they prove to be effective.

Conway pointed out that one benefit of having CMMI has been its ability to hasten the testing, learning, and change cycle and drive innovation into the marketplace relatively quickly. In his opinion, CMMI will be around for a long time because it has agreements in place in every state and community across the country and has people innovating in every state. One issue Banach identified, however, is that demonstrations are often viewed as ends in themselves. The point, he said, is not to have a hospice and concurrent care demonstration go on forever, but to create lasting change that may, in fact, require action by Congress.

Given the documented problems in coordinating the benefits provided by Medicare and Medicaid, Banach wondered what would happen if CMMI was given authority over all of Medicaid, not just the Medicaid side of PACE, and whether that would be a productive approach. Conway said CMMI's efforts are a work in progress, and one of the problems is that CMMI only has some authority over parts of Medicaid in a few states, not all of them. In his view, state-based innovation across Medicare and Medicaid that can flow seamlessly across state lines is needed to build momentum that will last from one administration to the next.

Conway noted that there is a provision in Title 11 of the Social Security Act that allows the government to use 1115 waivers to grant states great flexibility to customize their Medicaid programs to meet their state-based policy objectives.[37] States have used these waivers to expand coverage in certain cases and address delivery system reform objectives. That said, this is a politically fraught approach because of the magnitude of money involved—one waiver to one state could cost $5 to $10 billion over a 3-year period. Another type of waiver, the 1915 waiver,[38] allows for more tailored programs that are not as politically challenging, Conway added. Banach noted that a Medicare Advantage plan or ACO is free to provide a particular service under the terms of its contract. There is a difference between making a case-by-case determination, however, and requiring that a plan provide an actual benefit, such as food, transportation, or other non-medical service.

Whitlock raised a hypothetical situation in which an 80-year-old is taking care of her 80-year-old husband with Alzheimer's disease and doing so is hastening her decline. If Medicare allowed their primary care physician to order all of the services needed to keep them both in their home and out of nursing care and rewarded that physician for getting the husband into hospice in a timely manner that would lead to an alignment of desired outcomes and cost savings. The question he raised is how to get Medicare to start thinking that way under the current law. Today, Whitlock explained, Medicare's response to ordering Meals on Wheels would be that the physician is trying to create a food entitlement.

The Medicare–Medicaid dual-eligible demonstration, Medicare Advantage, and Medicaid Managed Care programs are starting to be creative about that type of approach, explained Harris. He also said Whitlock's example raised what he considers a big issue, which is that the system does not think of a husband and wife as a unit when it comes to Medicare, providing services, and keeping them both healthy and at home. That idea, he said, ties into the notion of providing caregiver support as part of the care plan for the person with serious illness. He noted that there are commercial plans that are considering making caregiver support available to employees as one component of workforce productivity initiatives.

---

[37] See https://www.ssa.gov/OP_Home/ssact/title11/1115A.htm (accessed January 22, 2018).
[38] See https://www.ssa.gov/OP_Home/ssact/title19/1915.htm (accessed January 23, 2018).

Harris commented that too often in policy discussions about adding non-medical benefits to Medicare to address social determinants of health, such as food or housing insecurity, the worry is that CMS will end up providing that benefit for everyone, which would bankrupt the system. Instead, he said, the conversation should be about defining those specific individuals—beneficiaries between 65 and 75 who have diabetes and COPD, for example—that would have lower health care costs if they had housing support and providing the benefit to that defined population. The key, he said, will be to build an evidence base that providing specific non-medical benefits to certain groups of beneficiaries will have a measurable effect on health outcomes and on the total cost of care. Otherwise, he added, there will be no support in Congress for scaling those types of benefits.

Harris noted that compared with other Organisation for Economic Co-operation and Development (OECD) countries, the United States spends far more on health care and far less on social services, although the combined totals are about the same (OECD, 2017). The difference is that other OECD countries are getting better health outcomes. In his mind, achieving that result in the United States would require aligning budgets across the various components of the U.S. Departments of Health and Human Services, Housing and Urban Development, Education, and perhaps others. That would be a massive undertaking, but it is not necessarily impossible, he said, and perhaps people should be thinking about how to make that happen. There was a time, for example, when states had the ability to combine Medicaid dollars with funds from other health-related social services agencies to invest in technology, and today there are programs that use Medicaid dollars to provide coordination to help people access existing housing benefits. Conway added that some states, including North Carolina, are using their waiver authorities to begin experiments at blending financing streams for medical and social services and perhaps demonstrate what is possible in that realm.

Allison Silvers from the Center to Advance Palliative Care pointed out one problem with that type of approach: there will be budgetary winners and losers, assuming the total pot of money will not grow. The politically tone-deaf answer to that issue, said Banach, is that it will require rationing of expensive services to make other services more available. Whitlock agreed with Banach and said that reality speaks to the scope of the challenge the nation faces as it tries to restructure its health care delivery and financing structures. Complicating the matter, he said, is the unrealistic expectation most Americans have about how they will age. Many believe they will have a long and healthy retirement, pass away in their own beds surrounded by loved ones, and never need serious illness care nor worry about how to pay for services outside of the purview of Medicare. In addition, many providers do not want to have the difficult conversations with patients and family members about what is appropriate for end-of-life care. Addressing those problems, he said, requires culture change, not new payment models.

Conway noted that the two biggest drivers of increasing medical costs, aside from the aging population, are hospital and pharmaceutical costs (Dieleman et al., 2017). Harris said he suspects that if a hospital or health system's financial arrangement gives it complete accountability for the total cost of care as well as flexibility on how it provides services, it would use some of those funds outside of the hospital or health care system in ways that would have a greater impact on improving health outcomes. At the same time, this would slow the growth of hospital-based health care costs. With respect to pharmaceutical costs, Harris believes that the amount of innovation in developing new therapies that is happening today will have the potential to slow the cost trajectory.

## Closing Thoughts

In her final comments to close out the workshop, Haiden Huskamp, 30th anniversary professor of health care policy at Harvard Medical School and co-chair of the workshop planning committee, referred to Meier's observation earlier in the day that the U.S. health care system is designed to get precisely the results that Americans currently experience. Huskamp noted that although there has been a tremendous amount of effort expended on redesigning the health care delivery system to produce better outcomes, care delivery redesign alone could only go so far. Huskamp pointed out that financing and payment strategies that support innovative care delivery models are crucial to their success and sustainability. "You can create the best program in the world, but if you cannot figure out how to keep it going because you cannot get the financing in order, where are you?" she asked. Huskamp noted the range of issues from workforce to quality measurement challenges faced by those who work to develop and implement financing approaches to support improved care for people facing serious illness.

In closing, Huskamp reminded participants of Senator Wyden's observation that they may currently be at an inflection point. She encouraged workshop participants to consider pursuing a parallel track: Work on short-term changes as Ling articulated earlier in the workshop, while continuing to focus on the long-term changes that are required to address the problems faced by couples such as the Bencivengas. The ultimate goal would be to advance both the care delivery and financing systems to enable the nation to meaningfully address the complex range of needs of people living with serious illness.

## REFERENCES

Aldridge, M. D., and A. S. Kelley. 2015. The myth regarding the high cost of end-of-life care. *American Journal of Public Health* 105(12):2411–2415.

BCBSMA (Blue Cross Blue Shield of Massachusetts). 2015. *More members to benefit from payment model that emphasizes quality of care innovative payment program will include Blue Cross PPO members in 2016.* http://newsroom.bluecrossma.com/2015-10-05-More-Members-To-Benefit-From-Payment-Model-That-Emphasizes-Quality-Of-Care-Innovative-payment-program-will-include-Blue-Cross-PPO-members-in-2016 (accessed April 19, 2018).

Center for Health Information and Analysis. 2017. *Annual report on the performance of the Massachusetts health care system.* http://archives.lib.state.ma.us/handle/2452/737375 (accessed April 19, 2018).

CMS (Centers for Medicare & Medicaid Services). 2017a. *Independence at home demonstration.* https://innovation.cms.gov/initiatives/independence-at-home (accessed January 24, 2018).

CMS. 2017b. *Medicare & home health care.* Baltimore, MD. https://www.medicare.gov/Pubs/pdf/10969-Medicare-and-Home-Health-Care.pdf (accessed April 19, 2018).

CMS. 2017c. *NHPCO facts and figures: Hospice care in America.* Alexandria, VA: National Hospice and Palliative Care Organization, March 2018. https://www.nhpco.org/sites/default/files/public/Statistics_Research/2017_Facts_Figures.pdf (accessed April 19, 2018).

CMS. 2018. *Shared savings program.* https://www.cms.gov/Medicare/Medicare-Fee-for-Service-Payment/sharedsavingsprogram/index.html?redirect=/sharedsavingsprogram/37e_Quality_Measures_Standards.asp#TopOfPage (accessed January 17, 2018).

Cubanski, J., T. Neuman, S. Griffin, and A. Damico. 2016. *Medicare spending at the end of life: A snapshot of beneficiaries who died in 2014 and the cost of their care.* https://www.kff.org/medicare/issue-brief/medicare-spending-at-the-end-of-life (accessed January 11, 2018).

Dieleman, J. L., E. Squires, A. L. Bui, M Campbell, A. Chaipin, H. Hamavid, C. Horst, Z. Li, T. Matyasz, A. Reynolds, N. Sadat, M. Schneider, and C. Murray. 2017. Factors associated with increases in U.S. health care spending, 1996–2013. *JAMA* 318(17):1668–1678.

Dumanovsky, T., R. Augustin, M. Rogers, K. Lettang, D. E. Meier, and R. S. Morrison. 2016. The growth of palliative care in U.S. hospitals: A status report. *Journal of Palliative Medicine* 19(1):8–15.

Gozalo, P., M. Plotzke, V. Mor, S. C. Miller, and J. M. Teno. 2015. Changes in Medicare costs with the growth of hospice care in nursing homes. *New England Journal of Medicine* 372(19):1823–1831.

Henry, S. L., E. Shen, A. Ahuja, M. K. Gould, and M. H. Kanter. 2016. The online personal action plan: A tool to transform patient-enabled preventive and chronic care. *American Journal of Preventive Medicine* 51(1):71–77.

HHS (U.S. Department of Health and Human Services). 2013. *45 CFR parts 147, 155, and 156 Patient Protection and Affordable Care Act; standards related to essential health benefits, actuarial value, and accreditation; Final Rule.* College Park, MD: National Archives and Records Administration: U.S. Department of Health and Human Services.

IOM (Institute of Medicine). 2003. *When children die: Improving palliative and end-of-life care for children and their families.* Washington, DC: The National Academies Press.

IOM. 2015. *Dying in America: Improving quality and honoring individual preferences near the end of life.* Washington, DC: The National Academies Press.

Jacobson, G., A. Damico, T. Neuman, and M. Gold. 2017. *Medicare Advantage 2017 spotlight: Enrollment market update.* http://files.kff.org/attachment/Issue-Brief-Medicare-Advantage-2017-Spotlight-Enrollment-Market-Update (accessed January 23, 2018).

Kaiser Permanente. 2013. "Complete care" improves patient outcomes: The Joint Commission Journal on Quality and Patient Safety praises Kaiser Permanente's Chronic Care Management Model. https://share.kaiserpermanente.org/article/complete-care-improves-patient-outcomes (accessed January 23, 2018).

Kelley, A. S., K. McGarry, S. Fahle, S. M. Marshall, Q. Du, and J. S. Skinner. 2013. Out-of-pocket spending in the last five years of life. *Journal of General Internal Medicine* 28(2):304–309.

MedPAC (Medicare Payment Advisory Committee). 2017. *March 2017 Report to the Congress: Medicare payment policy* 315–342. http://www.medpac.gov/docs/default-source/reports/mar17_medpac_ch12.pdf?sfvrsn=0 (accessed January 23, 2018).

Mor, V., O. Intrator, Z. Feng, and D. C. Grabowski. 2010. The revolving door of rehospitalization from skilled nursing facilities. *Health Affairs (Project HOPE)* 29(1):57–64.

NASEM (National Academies of Sciences, Engineering, and Medicine). 2017a. *Integrating the patient and caregiver voice into serious illness care: Proceedings of a workshop.* Washington, DC: The National Academies Press.

NASEM. 2017b. *Models and strategies to integrate palliative care principles into care for people with serious illness: Proceedings of a workshop.* Washington, DC: The National Academies Press.

OECD (Organisation for Economic Co-operation and Development). 2017. *Government at a glance 2017.* Paris: OECD Publishing. http://dx.doi.org/10.1787/gov_glance-2017-en (accessed January 23, 2018).

ProHEALTH. 2017. *Delivering home-based palliative care within an ACO.* https://www.accountablecarelc.org/sites/default/files/ACLC_CSB_ProHealth_Final.pdf (accessed March 5, 2018).

Rao, J. K., L. A. Anderson, F. C. Lin, and J. P. Laux. 2014. Completion of advance directives among U.S. consumers. *American Journal of Preventive Medicine* 46(1):65–70.

Sharp HealthCare. 2017. *Providing early palliative care interventions for patients with serious illness*. San Diego, CA: Sharp HealthCare. https://www.accountablecarelc.org/sites/default/files/ACLC_CSB_Sharp_Final.pdf (accessed March 5, 2018).

Song, Z., S. Rose, D. G. Safran, B. E. Landon, M. P. Day, and M. E. Chernew. 2014. Changes in health care spending and quality 4 years into global payment. *New England Journal of Medicine* 371(18):1704–1714.

Spence, M. M., J. K. Polzin, C. L. Weisberger, J. P. Martin, J. P. Rho, and G. H. Willick. 2011. Evaluation of a pharmacist-managed amiodarone monitoring program. *Journal of Managed Care & Specialty Pharmacy* 17(7):513–522.

Teno, J. M., P. L. Gozalo, J. P. W. Bynum, N. E. Leland, S. C. Miller, N. E. Morden, T. Scupp, D. C. Goodman, and V. Mor. 2013. Change in end-of-life care for Medicare beneficiaries: Site of death, place of care, and health care transitions in 2000, 2005, and 2009. *JAMA* 309(5):470–477.

The Economist Intelligence Unit. 2015. *The 2015 quality of death index: Ranking palliative care across the world*. The Economist. https://www.eiuperspectives.economist.com/sites/default/files/2015%20EIU%20Quality%20of%20Death%20Index%20Oct%2029%20FINAL.pdf (accessed January 29, 2018).

# Appendix A

# Statement of Task

An ad hoc committee will plan and host a 1-day public workshop that will examine how various financing and payment approaches can help support delivery of high-quality care for serious illness. The workshop will feature invited presentations and panel discussions on topics that may include

- Integrated financing models such as Medicare Advantage programs, Programs of All-Inclusive Care for the Elderly, and risk-based payment approaches such as accountable care organizations and bundled payments.
- Programs such as the Medicare hospice benefit, Medicare Home Health Care, Medicaid Home Health Care, and financing and payment methods for the dual-eligible population.
- Incorporation of performance metrics in payment models, such as pay-for-performance and performance incentives.
- Potential policy steps to address key gaps, challenges, and opportunities related to financing and payment models to support high-quality care for serious illness.

The planning committee will develop the agenda for the workshop, select speakers and discussants, and moderate the discussions. Proceedings of the presentations and discussions at the workshop will be prepared by a designated rapporteur in accordance with institutional guidelines.

# Appendix B

# Workshop Agenda

Financing and Payment Strategies to Support High-Quality Care for People with Serious Illness: A Workshop

Keck Center of the National Academies
500 Fifth Street, NW, Room 100
Washington, DC 20001

November 29, 2017

Workshop Objectives

- Explore innovative financing and payment strategies across a range of settings for people of all ages facing serious illness.
- Identify existing barriers to scale and spread of financing and payment innovations.
- Examine potential policy actions to address barriers to innovation.

**Wednesday, November 29, 2017**

8:00 am    **Registration and Breakfast**

8:30 am    **Welcome from the Roundtable on Quality Care for People with Serious Illness**
Leonard D. Schaeffer (*Chair*) and James A. Tulsky (*Vice Chair*)

**Overview of the Workshop**
Mark Ganz and Haiden Huskamp, Planning Committee Co-Chairs

**8:40 am**    **Session 1: Financing High-Quality Care for People with Serious Illness**

*Moderator: Haiden Huskamp, Ph.D., 30th Anniversary Professor of Health Care Policy, Harvard Medical School*

**Session 1A: Patient–Caregiver–Clinician Perspective**

Interview with a patient/family caregiver and his clinician.

*Interviewer: Patricia Bomba, M.D., Vice President and Medical Director, Geriatrics, Excellus BlueCross BlueShield*

Speakers:
- Ralph Bencivenga, Patient/Family Caregiver Perspective
- Bethann Scarborough, M.D., Associate Director of Ambulatory Services and Assistant Professor of Palliative Medicine, Icahn School of Medicine at Mount Sinai, Clinician Perspective

**9:20 am**    **Session 1B: Framing the Challenges and Opportunities for Financing and Payment Innovation**

Overview of the current financing landscape for care for people with serious illness, including the gaps, challenges, and opportunities; overarching framework of different payment models for people of all ages, all stages of serious illness.

*Moderator: Haiden Huskamp*

Speakers:
- David Stevenson, Ph.D., Associate Professor of Health Policy, Vanderbilt University School of Medicine
- Diane Meier, M.D., Director, Center to Advance Palliative Care

**Audience Q & A**

**10:15 am**    **Break**

**10:30 am  Session 2: Financing and Payment Innovations: Challenges, Impact, and Lessons Learned from Fee-for-Service and Value-Based Payment Arrangements**

This session will explore examples of challenges and opportunities for innovation in fee-for-service and value-based payment systems across a range of settings and patient populations. Speakers will discuss lessons learned from their efforts to implement innovative financing and payment arrangements and identify the key barriers to such innovation.

*Moderator: Harold L. Paz, M.D., Executive Vice President and Chief Medical Officer, Aetna*

Speakers:
- Richard Popiel, M.D., Executive Vice President and Chief Medical Officer, Cambia Health Solutions
- Jeanne Chirico, M.P.A., Vice President of Community Services for Lifetime Care and Director, Excellus BlueCross BlueShield CompassionNet Program
- David Debono, M.D., Medical Director, Oncology, Anthem, Inc.
- Shari Ling, M.D., Deputy Chief Medical Officer, Center for Clinical Standards and Quality, Centers for Medicare & Medicaid Services
- Robert L. Fine, M.D., Clinical Director, Office of Clinical Ethics and Palliative Care, Baylor Scott & White Health

**Panel Discussion/Audience Q & A**

**12:00 pm  Luncheon Keynote Speakers**

**12:00–12:45 pm**
Members of Congress have been invited to discuss the legislative and policy environment related to care for people with serious illness.

**U.S. Senator Ron Wyden (D-OR),** Ranking Member, Senate Committee on Finance
**U.S. Representative Phil Roe (R-TN),** Chair, House Committee on Veterans' Affairs

**Buffet Lunch**
**12:45–1:40 pm**

1:45 pm  **Session 3: Financing and Payment Innovations: Challenges, Impact, and Lessons Learned in Global Budgeting Arrangements**

This session will explore examples of challenges and opportunities for innovation in global budgeting arrangements across a range of settings and patient populations. Speakers will discuss lessons learned from their efforts to implement innovative financing and payment arrangements and identify the key barriers to such innovation.

*Moderator: Cheryl Phillips, M.D., President and CEO, SNP Alliance*

Speakers:
- Susan E. Wang, M.D., Regional Lead, Shared Decision-Making, Southern California Permanente Medical Group, Kaiser Permanente, and Annet Arakelian, Pharm.D., FCSHP, CPHQ, Executive Director, Medicare Strategy and Care Delivery, Kaiser Permanente
- Anna Gosline, M.P.H., Senior Director of Health Policy and Strategic Initiatives, Blue Cross Blue Shield of Massachusetts
- Vicki Jackson, M.D., Chief, Division of Palliative Care and Geriatric Medicine, Massachusetts General Hospital
- Gregory James, D.O., Senior Medical Director, OptumCare

**Panel Discussion/Audience Q & A**

APPENDIX B

**3:15 pm** **Break**

**3:30 pm** **Session 4A: Regulatory and Policy Changes to Ensure High-Quality Care for People of All Ages with Serious Illness**

Dr. Conway will share his insights and perspectives on policy and regulatory changes to ensure high-quality care for people with serious illness.

*Moderator: Mark Ganz, President and CEO, Cambia Health Solutions*

Keynote Presentation:
- Patrick Conway, M.D., President and CEO-Elect, Blue Cross Blue Shield of North Carolina

**3:50 pm** **Session 4B: Next Steps**

This session will focus on policy changes necessary at the federal and state levels to address barriers to financing and payment innovation to support high-quality care for people with serious illness.

*Moderator and Discussant: Patrick Conway*

Speakers:
- Edo Banach, J.D., President and CEO, National Hospice and Palliative Care Organization
- Julian Harris, M.D., M.B.A., President, CareAllies
- Rodney L. Whitlock, Ph.D., Vice President, Health Policy, ML Strategies

**Panel Discussion/Audience Q & A**

**5:15 pm** **Wrap-Up and Adjourn**
Mark Ganz and Haiden Huskamp